# Telomerase
## The Nectar of Immortality

by

Vivian

"Researchers have shown that secretions of the Skene's Glands contain an enzyme that extends the life of cells; hence female ejaculate has been called the nectar of youth or the enzyme of immortality. It is most probable that this enzyme is **Telomerase**, which decreases the ageing of cells."

*The Healing Power of the Sacred Woman: Health, Creativity, and Fertility for the Soul*
by Christine R. Page MD
Bear & Co (November 20, 2012)

# **Preface**

This small essay started as a compendium of notes on the female reproductive anatomy that grew into something bigger – a one hundred page collection of details relevant to the subject of a woman's body and how it is a pharmacologists delight. More to the point is the central theme of Telomerase as a life-generating enzyme – The Nectar of Immortality.

It is assumed that female architecture is understood by the casual reader - unfortunately it is not true. The details can be skipped without losing the essence but have been enclosed for easy reference.

The notes have been inserted verbatim to comprehend the intricate details and chemical compositions as well of 'generative fluids', for ant of a better term, available free for use if granted by the donor.

The subject is controversial, resisted tooth-and-nail by our male-dominated Judeo-Christian belief system and closely guarded by WICCANS who have, in the recent three decades, jealously let their secrets out in bits and pieces.

The style is direct – there has not been sufficient time to edit the compendium and no publisher was willing to touch this. Inserted are useful tips and discoveries – the discovery of female ejaculae or why it is no longer important to feed the male fetish and remove pubic hair.

As women come out of the closet, it is hoped this newfound discovery will not gather dust on the shelves but make us think, ponder and reflect.

Colloquial expressions to describe the anatomy have been used to make the compendium more entertaining rather than burden the user with drab medical terminology.

# **Star Tarot Card**

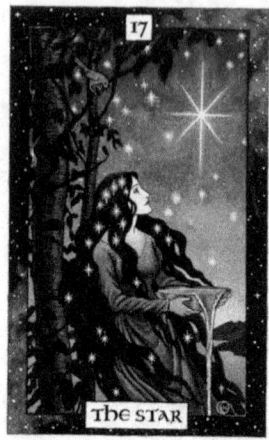

Star Card Symbols

Seven or eight stars, a kneeling woman (usually nude),
a pool of water, two urns.

## **Story**

On the bleak landscape where the Tower stood, the Fool
sits, empty, despairing. He hoped to find direction on
this spiritual journey, a path to his spiritual self, but
having just learned that most of his life was a lie, he now
feels lost.

Sitting on the cold stones, he gazes up at the night sky
wishing for some kind of guide.

And that is when he notices, nearby, a beautiful girl with
two water urns.

As he watches, she kneels by a pool of water illuminated
with reflected starlight. She empties the urns, one into
the pool, one onto the thirsty ground.

"What are you doing," he asks her.

She looks up at him, her eyes twinkling like stars. "I am refilling this pool, so that those who are thirsty may drink, and I am also watering the earth so that more fruit trees will grow to feed those who are hungry."

She nods back to a single fruit tree that stands nearby, a nightingale singing amid its branches.

**"Come," she invites. "Sate your hunger and quench your thirst."**

http://www.aeclectic.net/tarot/learn/meanings/star.shtml

# **Telomerase**

Telomerase, also called telomere terminal transferase, is a ribonucleoprotein that adds the polynucleotide "TTAGGG" to the 3' end of telomeres, which are found at the ends of eukaryotic chromosomes.

The human body is an organism formed by adding many organ systems together. Those organ systems are made of individual organs. Each organ contains tissues designed for specific functions like absorption and secretion. Tissues are made of cells that have joined together to perform those special functions. Each cell is then made of smaller components called organelles, one of which is called the nucleus.

The nucleus contains structures called chromosomes that are actually "packages" of all the genetic information that is passed from parents to their children.

The genetic information, or "genes," is really just a series of bases called Adenine (A), Guanine (G), Cytosine (C), and Thymine (T). These base pairs make up our cellular alphabet and create the sequences, or instructions needed to form our bodies.

To grow and age, our bodies must duplicate their cells. This process is called mitosis. Mitosis is a process that allows one "parent" cell to divide into two new "daughter" cells. During mitosis, cells make copies of their genetic material. Half of the genetic material goes to each new daughter cell.

To make sure that information is successfully passed from one generation to the next, each chromosome has a special protective cap called a telomere located at the end of its "arms." Telomeres are controlled by the presence of the enzyme telomerase.

A telomere is a repeating DNA sequence (for example, TTAGGG) at the end of the body's chromosomes. The telomere can reach a length of 15,000 base pairs. Telomeres function by preventing chromosomes from losing base pair sequences at their ends. They also stop chromosomes from fusing to each other.

Each time a cell divides, some of the telomere is lost (usually 25-200 base pairs per division). When the telomere becomes too short, the chromosome reaches a "critical length" and can no longer replicate. This means that a cell becomes "old" and dies by a process called apoptosis. Telomere activity is controlled by two mechanisms: erosion and addition. Erosion, as mentioned, occurs each time a cell divides. Addition is determined by the activity of telomerase.

Telomerase, also called telomere terminal transferase, is an enzyme made of protein and RNA subunits that elongates chromosomes by adding TTAGGG sequences to the end of existing chromosomes.

Telomerase is found in fetal tissues, adult germ cells, and also tumor cells. Telomerase activity is regulated during development and has a very low, almost undetectable activity in somatic (body) cells. Because these somatic cells do not regularly use telomerase, they age.

The result of aging cells is an aging body. If telomerase is activated in a cell, the cell will continue to grow and divide. This "immortal cell" theory is important in two areas of research: aging and cancer.

Cellular aging, or senescence, is the process by which a cell becomes old and dies. It is due to the shortening of chromosomal telomeres to the point that the chromosome reaches a critical length.

Cellular aging is analogous to a wind up clock. If the clock stays wound, a cell becomes immortal and constantly produces new cells. If the clock winds down, the cell stops producing new cells and dies.

Our cells are constantly aging. Being able to make the body's cells live forever certainly creates some exciting possibilities. Telomerase research could therefore yield important discoveries related to the aging process.

Cancer cells are a type of malignant cell. The malignant cells multiply until they form a tumor that grows uncontrollably. Telomerase has been detected in human cancer cells and is found to be 10-20 times more active than in normal body cells.

This provides a selective growth advantage to many types of tumors. If telomerase activity was to be turned off, then telomeres in cancer cells would shorten, just like they do in normal body cells. This would prevent the cancer cells from dividing uncontrollably in their early stages of development.

In the event that a tumor has already thoroughly developed, it may be removed and anti-telomerase therapy could be administered to prevent relapse. In essence, preventing telomerase from performing its function would change cancer cells from "immortal" to "mortal."

Knowing what we have just learned about telomeres and telomerase, it can be said that scientists are on the verge of discovering many of telomerase's secrets.

In the future, their research in the area of telomerase could uncover valuable information to combat aging, fight cancer, and even improve the quality of medical treatment in other areas such as skin grafts for burn victims, bone marrow transplants and heart disease.

# Protein Coding

## Telomerase Reverse Transcriptase (TERT)

TERT (Telomerase Reverse Transcriptase) is a Protein Coding gene.

Telomerase is a ribonucleoprotein polymerase that maintains telomere ends by addition of the telomere repeat TTAGGG.

The enzyme consists of a protein component with reverse transcriptase activity, encoded by this gene, and an RNA component which serves as a template for the telomere repeat.

Telomerase expression plays a role in cellular senescence, as it is normally repressed in postnatal somatic cells resulting in progressive shortening of telomeres.

Deregulation of telomerase expression in somatic cells may be involved in oncogenesis.

Studies in mice suggest that telomerase also participates in chromosomal repair, since de novo synthesis of telomere repeats may occur at double-stranded breaks.

Alternatively spliced variants encoding different isoforms of telomerase reverse transcriptase have been identified; the full-length sequence of some variants has not been determined.

Alternative splicing at this locus is thought to be one mechanism of regulation of telomerase activity.

Diseases associated with TERT include bone marrow failure, telomere-related, 1 and dyskeratosis congenita, autosomal recessive 4.

Among its related pathways are Apoptotic Pathways in Synovial Fibroblasts and Cell Cycle, Mitotic.

GO annotations related to this gene include protein homodimerization activity and telomerase activity.

## Genomic View for TERT Gene

Chr 5

**UCSC Golden Path with GeneCards custom track**
**Cytogenetic band:**
**5p15.33 by Ensembl 5p15.33 by Entrez Gene 5p15.33 by HGNC**

Telomerase is a ribonucleoprotein enzyme essential for the replication of chromosome termini in most eukaryotes.

Active in progenitor and cancer cells. Inactive, or very low activity, in normal somatic cells.

Catalytic component of the teleromerase holoenzyme complex whose main activity is the elongation of telomeres by acting as a reverse transcriptase that adds simple sequence repeats to chromosome ends by copying a template sequence within the RNA component of the enzyme.

Catalyzes the RNA-dependent extension of 3-chromosomal termini with the 6-nucleotide telomeric repeat unit, 5-TTAGGG-3.

The catalytic cycle involves primer binding, primer extension and release of product once the template boundary has been reached or nascent product translocation followed by further extension.

More active on substrates containing 2 or 3 telomeric repeats.

Telomerase activity is regulated by a number of factors including telomerase complex-associated proteins, chaperones and polypeptide modifiers. Telomerase plays important roles in aging and anti-apoptosis.

Telomerase is a ribonucleoprotein composed of an internal telomerase RNA template (TERC) and the enzyme, telomerase reverse transcriptase (TERT).

Telomerase adds small repeat sequences of DNA (TTAGGG) to the end of chromosomes - multiple repeats of this hexanucleotide sequence over a 5kb span are known as a telomere. During normal cellular replication, telomeres are eroded and thus protect the coding sequences of the DNA. The erosion of telomeric sequences is thought

to form the basis of the cellular clock which eventually signals for the cell to exit the cell cycle and undergo senescence. Expression of telomerase is low in most normal cells although it is thought to be active in embryonic cells and some rapidly dividing cells of the immune system.

Overexpression of telomerase is key component of the transformation process in many malignant cancer cells.

*www.genecards.org/cgi-bin/carddisp.pl?gene=TERT*

# **Altar**

The mons pubis or The Altar and known specifically in females as the mons Venus or mons veneris), is a rounded mass of fatty tissue found over the pubic symphysis of the pubic bones. The Altar forms the anterior portion of the vulva.

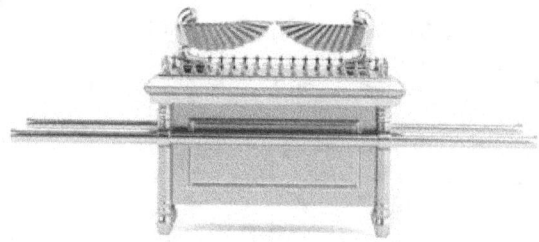

It divides into the labia majora (literally "larger lips"), on either side of the furrow known as the pudendal cleft, which surrounds the labia minora, clitoris, urethra, vaginal opening, and other structures of the vulval vestibule.

The size of the Altar varies with the level of hormone and body fat, and it is more apparent in females.

After puberty, it generally becomes covered with pubic hair and enlarged. The fatty tissue of the Altar is sensitive to estrogen, causing a distinct mound to form with the onset of puberty. This pushes the forward portion of the labia majora out and away from the pubic bone.

The Altar is also termed as mons, mons veneris, or pubic mound. It is the fat pad covering on the pubic bone which segments to create The Outer Gate.

The main purpose of The Altar is to give cushioning and protection to the pubic You do not have access to view this node, mainly during intercourse and also protect the bones and tissues lying beneath.

In the beginning the Altar does not have any hair but as a woman reaches puberty the Altar too becomes thick and is covered with thick pubic hair. The anterior part of vulva is formed by The Altar.

The Altar segments into the Outer Gate also known as larger lips on both the sides of furrow and is termed as cleft of venus which also encircles labia minor, vaginal opening and clitoris along with other parts of the vulval vestibule.

The fatty tissue which mostly composes the Altar or mons veneris is highly sensitive towards, estrogen and hence forms a visible mound when women reache puberty.

Due to this the labia majora part is pushed forward and is placed distant from pubic You do not have access to view this node.

During the intercourse, the body experiences motion on the genital areas which can cause injury to the delicate parts. Similarly, other reasons can too cause injury to this part and hence The Altar is located there to serve as the security pad for protecting this organ from any harm.

Apart from this, the Altar also assists in stimulating olfactory aromas that enhances the sexual attractiveness. Sebaceous and sweat glands are present inside the Altar that creates sexually appealing smell to stimulate arousal.

.

# **Threshold**

The vulva is the collective name for the external female genitalia in the pubic region, including the labia, cherry, and urethral and vaginal openings. These organs work together to support urination and sexual reproduction.

The exterior of the vulva begins as a mound of skin-covered adipose known as the Altar that arises from the skin covering the pubis bone in the pubic region.

As it continues inferiorly, the Altar divides laterally into the two parallel Outer Gate. The Outer Gate are wide folds of skin and adipose that rise beyond the Altar and surround the pudendal cleft, a deep vertical furrow in the center of the vulva.

Both the Altar and Outer Gate are covered in pubic hair following puberty and serve to protect the delicate structures of the vulva found in the pudendal cleft.

Medial to the Outer Gate in the pudendal cleft are a pair of hairless folds of skin known as the Inner Gate. Compared to the Outer Gate, the Inner Gate are much thinner and longer structures, extending from the pudendal cleft beyond the top of the Outer Gate. Nestled within the Inner Gate from anterior to posterior are the cherry, the external urethral orifice, and the vaginal orifice.

The Inner Gate meet anteriorly just above the cherry at a small fold of tissue known as the prepuce (or clitoral hood) and merge posteriorly just below the vaginal orifice.

The cherry is a small mass of highly sensitive erectile tissue that receives mechanical stimulation during sexual contact and transmits sensations of sexual pleasure to the brain.

Thousands of touch and pressure sensitive nerve endings are packed into the cherry, making it the most sensitive erogenous organ of the vulva.

During sexual stimulation, erectile tissue in the cherryfills with blood, causing it to enlarge, extend beyond the prepuce, and become more susceptible to stimulation.

The cherryalso extends into the internal tissues of the vulva and is sensitive to mechanical stimulus inside of the vagina as well.

The external urethral orifice is a small hole in the vulva surrounded by a ring of slightly raised skin. It provides the connection for the urethra to the body's exterior and permits the release of urine during the process of urination. Pathogenic bacteria present on the skin covering the vulva may enter the urethra through the external urethral orifice, resulting in urinary tract infections.

The vaginal orifice is the external connection between the vagina and the body's exterior. It is much larger and more elastic than the external urethral orifice and allows for penetration during sex.

# **Temple**

The temple is an elastic, muscular tube connecting the cervix of the uterus to the vulva and exterior of the body. The temple is located in the pelvic body cavity posterior to the urinary bladder and anterior to the rectum.

Measuring around 3 inches in length and less than an inch in diameter, the temple stretches to become several inches longer and many inches wider during sexual intercourse and childbirth. The inner surface of the temple is folded to provide greater elasticity and to increase friction during sexual intercourse.

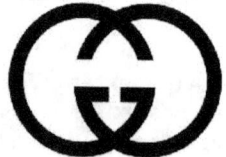

The inner lining of the temple is made of non-keratinized stratified squamous epithelial tissue. This tissue provides protection from friction to the underlying layers of the temple.

Watery secretions produced by the temple epithelium lubricate the temple and have an acidic pH to prevent the growth of bacteria and yeast.

The acidic pH also makes the temple an inhospitable environment for sperm, which has resulted in males producing alkaline seminal fluid to neutralize the acid and improve the survival of sperm.

Deep to the epithelial layer is the lamina propria, a layer of connective tissue with many elastin fibers that allow the temple to stretch.

A layer of smooth muscle tissue located deep to the lamina propria allows the temple to expand and contract during sexual intercourse and childbirth.

Surrounding the smooth muscle is the outermost layer of the temple known as the tunica externa. The tunica externa is a layer of dense irregular connective tissue that forms the outer protective shell of the temple.

During sexual intercourse, the temple functions as the receptacle till the uterus and fallopian tubes. The elastic structure of the temple allows it to stretch in both length and diameter.

# **Cherry**

The cherry is a small projection of erectile tissue in the vulva of the female reproductive system. It contains thousands of nerve endings that make it an extremely sensitive organ. Touch stimulation of the nerve endings in the cherry produces sensations of sexual pleasure. The cherry is structurally and functionally homologous to the penis of the male reproductive system, except that the cherry does not contain the urethra and plays no role in urination.

The cherry is located within the vulva at the anterior intersection of the labia minora. It is shaped like a wishbone.

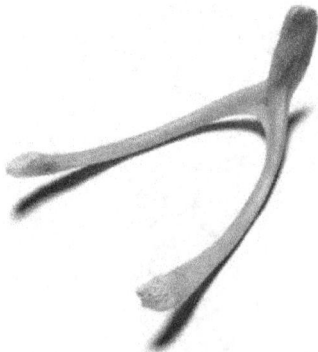

[ wishes granted ]

It is vaguely cylindrical in shape and usually just a centimeter or two in length, although its size may vary greatly in individuals.

The prepuce, or hood, of the cherry is a small fold of skin that covers and protects the cherry anteriorly; the labia majora and labia minora surround and protect it in all other directions.

The cherry can be divided into three major regions: the glans, body, and crura.

Under the surface of the skin, two legs of erectile tissue known as the crura fan out to support the exterior structures of the cherry and attach to the underlying tissues.

Extending from the crura is the body, the main cylindrical region of the cherry, which contains two columns of the erectile tissue. Blood filling the hollow chambers of the erectile tissue allows the cherry to grow in size and harden during sexual stimulation.

Finally, the glans forms the pointed tip of the cherry extending outward from the body and beyond the prepuce that covers the rest of the cherry.

Thousands of touch and pressure sensitive nerve endings are found throughout the cherry. Nerve endings in the body and glans are sensitive to direct touch and pressure stimulation from outside of the body while the nerve endings of the crus are sensitive to stimulation from within the temple. The stimulation of the clitoral nerve endings is responsible for the majority of sexual pleasure and sensation in the female body.

# **Outer Gate**

The Outer Gate is formed by a pair of rounded folds of skin and adipose that are part of the external female genitalia. Their function is to cover and protect the inner, more delicate and sensitive structures of the vulva, such as the Inner gate, cherry, pee-hole and Temple.

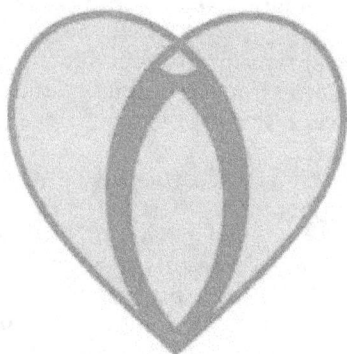

The Outer Gate is located in the pubic region on the surface of the body lateral to the Inner Gate, Cherry and the Temple.

They arise gradually from the skin of the pelvis and extend the Altar beyond the pelvic bones to the anus. Adipose tissue deep to the skin supports the Outer Gate and provides cushioning and flexibility to the pubic region.

The Outer Gate form the lateral borders of the pudendal cleft, the vertical fissure of the vulva. Anterior to the pudendal cleft, they join to form the anterior commissure of the Outer Gate, just inferior to the Altar. On the posterior end, the Outer Gate gradually merge with the surrounding skin in the perineal region at their posterior commissure.

The major function of the Outer Gate is protection of the softer tissues of the vulva.

Unlike the inner structures of the vulva, the Outer Gate contains Candy Floss to protect the rest of the vulva from mechanical stress and friction.

The adipose tissue of the Outer Gate also helps to cushion the vulva from exterior stresses. Many exocrine glands are associated with the hair follicles of Outer Gate, including apocrine sudoriferous glands, eccrine sudoriferous glands, and sebaceous glands. Eccrine sweat glands assist in thermoregulation by producing watery sweat, while sebaceous glands produce oil to lubricate the hair shafts and skin.

Apocrine sweat glands produce a fatty secretion that is consumed by bacteria living on the skin, producing a particular form of body odor. It is believed that the odor produced by apocrine sweat glands once acted as a pheromone to attract mates.

.

# **Inner Gate**

The lInner Gate is formed by a pair of thin cutaneous folds that form part of the vulva, or external female genitalia. They function as protective structures that surround the clitoris, urinary orifice, and vaginal orifice.

The Inner Gate is found within the vulva inferior to the Altar and medial to the Outer Gate within the pudendal cleft.

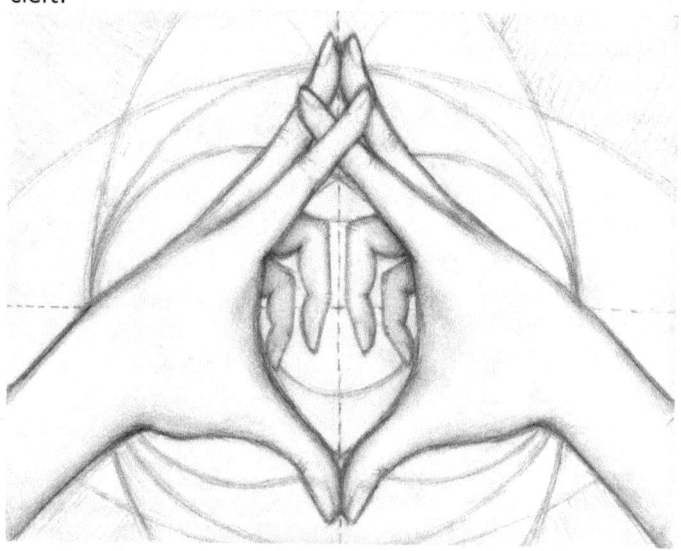

They extend from the floor of the pudendal cleft to the top of the Outer Gate or beyond, depending on the individual.

In fact, the Inner Gate show a considerable amount of variation in length, width, shape, and pigmentation between individuals.

Unlike the surrounding the Altar and Outer Gate, the Inner Gate is covered with hairless skin and contains very little adipose tissue.

At their anterior end they meet at the hood, or prepuce, where they surround the lateral sides of the clitoris.

From the hood, the Inner Gate extend inferiorly toward the anus, where they gradually decrease in size before merging with the skin of the perineum.

The middle region of the Inner Gate covers and protects the urethral orifice and vaginal orifice from the exterior environment.

The Inner Gate is made of several distinct layers of tissue. The outermost layer is made of non-keratinized stratified squamous epithelium continuous with the surrounding skin.

The lack of keratin makes the Inner Gate less tough and waterproof than the surrounding skin, but also makes them smoother and softer. Deep to the epithelium is a layer of fibrous connective tissue continuous with the dermis of the skin.

Collagen and elastin protein fibers present in the connective tissues provide strength and elasticity to the Inner Gate, while vascular and nervous tissues support the cells of the outer epithelial layer.

Blood flowing through many tiny capillaries in the connective tissue layer gives the Inner Gate their pinkish color. Many sebaceous glands are also present in the connective tissue and extend to the surface of the Inner Gate via ducts.

Sebum, or oil, produced by the sebaceous glands coats the surface of the Inner Gate to lubricate and protect the underlying tissues.

# **Nectar of Immortality**

According to Dr Christine R Page in her book 'Healing Power', Telomerase is produced by clitoral orgasm.

The clitoral organ system actually surrounds the temple, urethra and anus. Rather than thinking of an orgasm as "vaginal" or "clitoral", it makes more sense to think of the nectar which comes out after the act.

Sigmund Freud made a pronouncement that the "mature" woman has orgasms only when her temple, but not her cherry, is stimulated — this is commonly referred to as the "clitoral orgasm".

The emphasis on stimulation from penetration made the man's penis central to a woman's sexual satisfaction.

It is important to emphasize that Freud did not base his theory upon a study of woman's anatomy, but rather upon his assumptions of woman as inferior to men.

Back to the basics, stimulating the cherry and pressure in or around the temple can cause pelvic fullness and body tension to build up to a peak.

During sexual excitement, the cherry swells and changes position. The blood vessels through the whole pelvic area also swell – to cause engorgement and a feeling of fullness and sexual sensitivity.

The inner temple lips swell and change shape, and the temple balloons upward, causing the uterus to shift position.

Orgasm is the point at which all the tension is suddenly released in a series of involuntary and pleasurable muscular contractions in the temple and uterus.

The clitoral orgasm can be stimulated in a number of different ways — by rubbing, sucking, body pressure, or using a vibrator.

Although some women touch the glans of the cherry to become aroused, for others it can be so sensitive that direct touching hurts, even with lubrication.

Also, focusing directly on the cherry for a long time may cause the pleasurable sensations to disappear.

Your cherry can also be stimulated during sexual intercourse, most often with the woman on top — this happens when the cherry is rubbed against the man's pubic bone.

It can also be achieved when the man is on top if the man positions himself high enough so that his pubic bone presses against his partner's clitoral area.

You or your partner can also stimulate your cherry with fingers during intercourse to help bring you to orgasm.

Aside from clitoral stimulation, it is important to remember another major organ involved with orgasm — the brain! Emotions, perceptions, memories, and senses determine how we experience sex, rather than past experiences or physical appearance alone.

Mental (cortical) stimulation, where the imagination stimulates the brain, can actually help set off an orgasm. Relaxing and concentrating on sensations (rather than worrying about how you're doing) can help your brain process your pleasure.

Overall, orgasms are a very individualistic thing — there is no one correct pattern of sexual response. Whatever works, feels good, and makes you feel more alive and connected with your body are what count.

This nectar "release" is entirely unrelated to "templel" secretions, who's primary, but not exclusive purpose is the lubrication of the temple.

While there have been numerous claims of vast quantities of liquid expelled during ejaculation, all fail to offer a biologically compelling explanation as to the source, or reservoir used to store or produce such copious supplies of juices.

Regardless of the true quantity, it is a fact, that it is possible for some women to expel (or ejaculate) nectar.

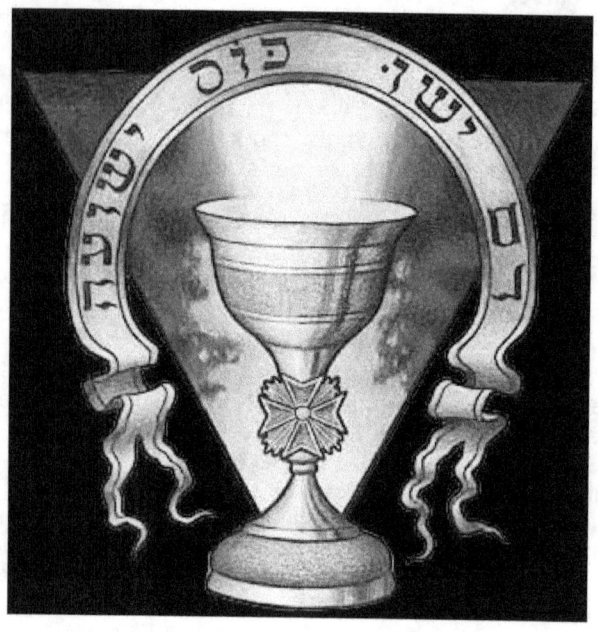

# Skene's Gland

The Skene's gland is embedded in the wall of the urethra, and can be indirectly felt through the upper temple wall, 2- 3" from the entrance of the temple.

For years the standard explanation was that the stuff was urine squeezed out of the bladder or urethra during the state of heightened muscle tension that accompanies orgasm.

But conventional wisdom has shifted over the past two decades, and most sex therapists now seem to think the discharge is more than plain old stress incontinence.

One thing that distinguishes nectar from urine is that it contains elevated levels of two proteins, prostate-specific antigen (PSA) and prostate-specific acid phosphatase (PSAP).

The emerging consensus, in fact, is that the paraurethral glands, which run more or less parallel to the urethra, are the "female prostate." Orgasm may cause these glands to empty out. Some think female ejaculate consists solely of discharge from the paraurethral glands, others that it's a mix of glandular secretions and urine

Both these propositions are questionable. According to Milan Zaviacic, a pathologist who has examined the female prostate on numerous occasions during autopsies, the gland is located at the site commonly believed to be the G-spot in women.

Even in cases where the female prostate and the G-spot coincide, no one has persuasively shown how that would account for the intense sensations associated with the G-spot--for example, that the female prostate is richly supplied with nerve endings.

The outer third of the templecanal does have plenty of nerve endings, but as far as we know they're not concentrated at a particular location.

Zaviacic goes on to say that "the type of the female prostate," found in 66 percent of women and located further down the urethra than the G-spot is supposed to be, "is a newly identified female erogenous zone important to coital female orgasm"--in short, he's still convinced the gland is sensitive to sexual stimulation, wherever it is.

Zaviacic cowrote a paper on the subject with Richard Ablin, who discovered PSA, and Edward Eichel, a therapist who advocates the "coital alignment technique" (CAT), a variation on the missionary position that supposedly makes it easier for the woman to come.

Eichel has described CAT as the "new intercourse," and says it works in part because it stimulates the female prostate. Many women would welcome any improvement on the dismal sexual technique of the average male, but we still don't have a convincing account of how the female prostate can produce sexual sensations

Zaviacic hasn't done any special investigation of the gland's innervation.

Although the ability of the female to ejaculate depends on a number of factors, it must be recognized that it is not for everyone. The effort to release Nectar is detailed, complex and requires sensitivity of the fingertips and loads of experience.

One of the safest ways determined by experienced practitioners of this art is to lie on your stomach and gently stimulate the cherry by embedding it between the forefingers of each hand.

Great care has to be taken not to damage the cherry by gently moving your hips in an undulating manner to get the maximum control on the time of release.

The problem with nectar is that on contact with an atom of oxygen, it is only partially effective i.e it becomes an "impure" or "contaminated" form of nectar, which may or may not give the results desired.

It is suggested that the person who wishes to avail of the benefits of nectar may directly lie down in close proximity to get the full stream of the precious stream for maximum effect. It is for the same reason that it cannot be bottled or stored.

# **DMT**

N,N-Dimethyltryptamine (DMT or N,N-DMT) is a psychedelic compound of the tryptamine family. It is a structural analog of serotonin and melatonin and a functional analog of other psychedelic tryptamines such as 4-AcO-DMT, 5-MeO-DMT, 5-HO-DMT, psilocybin (4-PO-DMT), and psilocin (4-HO-DMT).

It is consumed by indigenous Amazonian Amerindian cultures through the consumption of ayahuasca for divinatory and healing purposes.

Dimethyltryptamine is an indole alkaloid derived from the shikimate pathway. Its biosynthesis is relatively simple and summarized in the picture to the left. In plants, the parent amino acid L-tryptophan is produced endogenously where in animals L-tryptophan is an essential amino acid coming from diet.

No matter the source of L-tryptophan, the biosynthesis begins with its decarboxylation by an aromatic amino acid decarboxylase (AADC) enzyme (step 1). The resulting decarboxylated tryptophan analog is tryptamine. Tryptamine then undergoes a transmethylation (step 2): the enzyme indolethylamine-N-methyltransferase (INMT) catalyzes the transfer of a methyl group from cofactor S-adenosyl-methionine (SAM), via nucleophilic attack, to tryptamine.

This reaction transforms SAM into S-adenosylhomocysteine (SAH), and gives the intermediate product N-methyltryptamine (NMT).[17][18] NMT is in turn transmethylated by the same process (step 3) to form the end product N,N-dimethyltryptamine.

Tryptamine transmethylation is regulated by two products of the reaction: SAH, and DMT were shown ex vivo to be among the most potent inhibitors of rabbit INMT activity.

This transmethylation mechanism has been repeatedly and consistently proven by radiolabeling of SAM methyl group with carbon-14 (14C-CH3)SAM).

## Evidence in mammals

Published in Science in 1961, Julius Axelrod found an N-methyltransferase enzyme capable of mediating biotransformation of tryptamine into DMT in a rabbit's lung.

This finding initiated a still ongoing scientific interest in endogenous DMT production in humans and other mammals. From then on, two major complementary lines of evidence have been investigated: localisation and further characterization of the N-methyltransferase enzyme, and analytical studies looking for endogenously produced DMT in body fluids and tissues.

In 2013 researchers first reported DMT in the pineal gland. In the popular drug culture, this has been expanded to an assertion that it occurs in the human pineal gland, and is released at or shortly before death, but this conjecture has not yet been scientifically verified.

A study published in 2014 reported the biosynthesis of N,N-dimethyltryptamine (DMT) in the human melanoma cell line SK-Mel-147 including details on its metabolism by peroxidases.

In a 2014 paper a group first demonstrated the immunomodulatory potential of DMT and 5-MeO-DMT through the Sigma-1 receptor of human immune cells.

This immunomodulatory activity may contribute to significant anti-inflammatory effects and tissue regeneration.

# **INMT**

Before techniques of molecular biology were used to localize indolethylamine N-methyltransferase (INMT), characterization and localization went on a par.

Samples of the biological material where INMT is hypothesized to be active are subject to enzyme assay. Those enzyme assays are performed either with a radiolabeled methyl donor like (14C-CH3)SAM to which known amounts of unlabeled substrates like tryptamine are added or with addition of a radiolabeled substrate like (14C)NMT to demonstrate in vivo formation.

As qualitative determination of the radioactively tagged product of the enzymatic reaction is sufficient to characterize INMT existence and activity (or lack of), analytical methods used in INMT assays are not required to be as sensitive as those needed to directly detect and quantify the minute amounts of endogenously formed DMT (see DMT subsection below).

The essentially qualitative method thin layer chromatography (TLC) was thus used in a vast majority of studies. Also, robust evidence that INMT can catalyze transmethylation of tryptamine into NMT and DMT could be provided with reverse isotope dilution analysis coupled to mass spectrometry for human lung during the early 1970s.

Selectivity rather than sensitivity proved to be an Achilles' heel for some TLC methods with the discovery in 1974–1975 that incubating rat blood cells or brain tissue with (14C-CH3)SAM and NMT as substrate mostly yields tetrahydro-β-carboline derivatives, and negligible amounts of DMT in brain tissue.

It is indeed simultaneously realized that the TLC methods used thus far in almost all published studies on INMT and DMT biosynthesis are incapable to resolve DMT from those tetrahydro-β-carbolines.

These findings are a blow for all previous claims of evidence of INMT activity and DMT biosynthesis in avian and mammalian brain, including in vivo, as they all relied upon use of the problematic TLC methods.

Their validity is doubted in replication studies that make use of improved TLC methods, and fail to evidence DMT-producing INMT activity in rat and human brain tissues.

Published in 1978, the last study attempting to evidence in vivo INMT activity and DMT production in brain with TLC methods finds biotransformation of radiolabeled tryptamine into DMT to be real but "insignificant".

Capability of the method used in this latter study to resolve DMT from tetrahydro-β-carbolines is questioned.

To localize INMT, a qualitative leap is accomplished with use of modern techniques of molecular biology, and of immunohistochemistry. In humans, a gene encoding INMT is determined to be located on chromosome 7.

Northern blot analyses reveal INMT messenger RNA (mRNA) to be highly expressed in rabbit lung, and in human thyroid, adrenal gland, and lung.

Intermediate levels of expression are found in human heart, skeletal muscle, trachea, stomach, small intestine, pancreas, testis, prostate, placenta, lymph node, and spinal cord.

Low to very low levels of expression are noted in rabbit brain and human thymus, liver, spleen, kidney, colon, ovary, and bone marrow.

INMT mRNA expression is absent in human peripheral blood leukocytes, whole brain, and in tissue from 7 specific brain regions (thalamus, subthalamic nucleus, caudate nucleus, hippocampus, amygdala, substantia nigra, and corpus callosum).

Immunohistochemistry showed INMT to be present in large amounts in glandular epithelial cells of small and large intestines. In 2011, immunohistochemistry revealed the presence of INMT in primate nervous tissue including retina, spinal cord motor neurons, and pineal gland.

# Endogenous DMT

The first claimed detection of mammalian endogenous DMT was published in June 1965: German researchers F. Franzen and H. Gross report to have evidenced and quantified DMT, along with its structural analog bufotenin (5-HO-DMT), in human blood and urine.

In an article published four months later, the method used in their study was strongly criticized, and the credibility of their results challenged.

Few of the analytical methods used prior to 2001 to measure levels of endogenously formed DMT had enough sensitivity and selectivity to produce reliable results. Gas chromatography, preferably coupled to mass spectrometry (GC-MS), is considered a minimum requirement.

A study published in 2005 implements the most sensitive and selective method ever used to measure endogenous DMT:[46] liquid chromatography-tandem mass spectrometry with electrospray ionization (LC-ESI-MS/MS) allows for reaching limits of detection (LODs) 12 to 200 fold lower than those attained by the best methods employed in the 1970s.

## Physical and Chemical

DMT is commonly handled and stored as a fumarate, as other DMT acid salts are extremely hygroscopic and will not readily crystallize.

Its freebase form, although less stable than DMT fumarate, is favored by recreational users choosing to vaporize the chemical as it has a lower boiling point.

In contrast to DMT's base, its salts are water-soluble. DMT in solution degrades relatively quickly and should be stored protected from air, light, and heat in a freezer.

# 5-MeO-DMT

5-MeO-DMT, a psychedelic drug structurally similar to N,N-DMT, is sometimes referred to as DMT through abbreviation. As a white, crystalline solid, it is also similar in appearance to DMT. However, it is considerably more potent (5-MeO-DMT typical vaporized dose: 5–20 mg), and care should be taken to clearly differentiate between the two drugs to avoid accidental overdose.

## Pharmacokinetics

DMT peak level concentrations (Cmax) measured in whole blood after intramuscular (IM) injection (0.7 mg/kg, n = 11)[54] and in plasma following intravenous (IV) administration (0.4 mg/kg, n = 10)[55] of fully psychedelic doses are in the range of ≈14 to 154 µg/L and 32 to 204 µg/L, respectively.

The corresponding molar concentrations of DMT are therefore in the range of 0.074–0.818 µM in whole blood and 0.170–1.08 µM in plasma. However, several studies have described active transport and accumulation of DMT into rat and dog brain following peripheral administration.

Similar active transport, and accumulation processes likely occur in human brain and may concentrate DMT in brain by several-fold or more (relatively to blood), resulting in local concentrations in the micromolar or higher range.

Such concentrations would be commensurate with serotonin brain tissue concentrations, which have been consistently determined to be in the 1.5-4 µM range.

Closely coextending with peak psychedelic effects, mean time to reach peak concentrations (Tmax) was determined to be 10–15 minutes in whole blood after IM injection and 2 minutes in plasma after IV administration.

When taken orally mixed in an ayahuasca decoction, and in freeze-dried ayahuasca gel caps, DMT Tmax is considerably delayed: 107.59 ± 32.5 minutes,[63] and 90–120 minutes,[64] respectively.

## Pharmacodynamics

DMT binds non-selectively with affinities < 0.6 µM to the following serotonin receptors: 5-HT1A, 5-HT1B, 5-HT1D, 5-HT2A, 5-HT2B, 5-HT2C, 5-HT6 and 5-HT7.

An agonist action has been determined at 5-HT1A, 5-HT2A and 5-HT2C. Of special interest will be the determination of its efficacy at human 5-HT2B receptor as two in vitro assays evidenced DMT's high affinity for this receptor: 0.108 µM[68] and 0.184 µM.

This may be of importance because chronic or frequent uses of serotonergic drugs showing preferential high affinity and clear agonism at 5-HT2B receptor have been linked to valvular heart disease.

It has also been shown to possess affinity for the dopamine D1, α1-adrenergic, α2-adrenergic, imidazoline-1, and sigma-1 (σ1) receptors. Converging lines of evidence established activation of the σ1 receptor at concentrations of 50–100 µM.

It has also been shown in vitro to be a substrate for the cell-surface serotonin transporter (SERT) and the intracellular vesicular monoamine transporter 2 (VMAT2), inhibiting SERT-mediated serotonin uptake in human platelets at an average concentration of 4.00 ± 0.70 µM and VMAT2-mediated serotonin uptake in vesicles (of army worm Sf9 cells) expressing rat VMAT2 at an average concentration of 93 ± 6.8 µM.

# **DMT : Psychedelic Effects**

As with other so-called "classical hallucinogens", a large part of DMT psychedelic effects can be attributed to a functionally selective activation of the 5-HT2A receptor.

DMT concentrations eliciting 50% of its maximal effect (half maximal effective concentration = EC50 or Kact) at the human 5-HT2A receptor in vitro are in the 0.118–0.983 µM range.

This range of values coincides well with the range of concentrations measured in blood and plasma after administration of a fully psychedelic dose.

As DMT has been shown to have slightly better efficacy (EC50) at human serotonin 2C receptor than at the 2A receptor, 5-HT2C is also likely implicated in DMT's overall effects. Other receptors, such as 5-HT1A σ1, may also play a role.

In 2009, it was hypothesized that DMT may be an endogenous ligand for the σ1 receptor. The concentration of DMT needed for σ1 activation in vitro (50–100 µM) is similar to the behaviorally active concentration measured in mouse brain of approximately 106 µM which is minimally 4 orders of magnitude higher than the average concentrations measured in rat brain tissue or human plasma under basal conditions, so σ1 receptors are likely to be activated only under conditions of high local DMT concentrations.

If DMT is stored in synaptic vesicles, such concentrations might occur during vesicular release.

To illustrate, while the average concentration of serotonin in brain tissue is in the 1.5-4 µM range, the concentration of serotonin in synaptic vesicles was measured at 270 mM.

Following vesicular release, the resulting concentration of serotonin in the synaptic cleft, to which serotonin receptors are exposed, is estimated to be about 300 µM.

Thus, while in vitro receptor binding affinities, efficacies, and average concentrations in tissue or plasma are useful, they are not likely to predict DMT concentrations in the vesicles or at synaptic or intracellular receptors.

Under these conditions, notions of receptor selectivity are moot, and it seems probable that most of the receptors identified as targets for DMT participate in producing its **psychedelic effects**.

DMT is produced in many species of plants often in conjunction with its close chemical relatives 5-MeO-DMT and bufotenin (5-OH-DMT). DMT-containing plants are commonly used in South American shamanic practices.

It is usually one of the main active constituents of the drink ayahuasca; however, ayahuasca is sometimes brewed with plants that do not produce DMT. It occurs as the primary psychoactive alkaloid in several plants including Mimosa tenuiflora, Diplopterys cabrerana, and Psychotria viridis.

DMT is found as a minor alkaloid in snuff made from Virola bark resin in which 5-MeO-DMT is the main active alkaloid. DMT is also found as a minor alkaloid in bark, pods, and beans of Anadenanthera peregrina and Anadenanthera colubrina used to make Yopo and Vilca snuff in which bufotenin is the main active alkaloid. **Psilocin**, an active chemical in many psychedelic mushrooms, is structurally similar to DMT.

DMT can produce powerful psychedelic experiences including intense visuals, euphoria and hallucinations.
DMT is generally not active orally unless it is combined with a monoamine oxidase inhibitor (MAOI) such as a reversible inhibitor of monoamine oxidase A (RIMA), for example, harmaline.

Without an MAOI, the body quickly metabolizes orally administered DMT, and it therefore has no hallucinogenic effect unless the dose exceeds monoamine oxidase's metabolic capacity.

Other means of ingestion such as vaporizing, injecting, or insufflating the drug can produce powerful hallucinations for a short time (usually less than half an hour), as the DMT reaches the brain before it can be metabolized by the body's natural monoamine oxidase.

Taking a MAOI prior to vaporizing or injecting DMT prolongs and potentiates the effects.

DMT is broken down by the enzyme monoamine oxidase through a process called deamination, and is quickly inactivated orally unless combined with a monoamine oxidase inhibitor (MAOI).

The traditional South American beverage ayahuasca, or yage, is derived by boiling the ayahuasca vine (Banisteriopsis caapi) with leaves of one or more plants containing DMT, such as Psychotria viridis, Psychotria carthagenensis, or Diplopterys cabrerana The Ayahuasca vine contains harmala alkaloids, highly active reversible inihibitors of monoamine oxidase A (RIMAs), rendering the DMT orally active by protecting it from deamination.

A variety of different recipes are used to make the brew depending on the purpose of the ayahuasca session or local availability of ingredients. Two common sources of DMT in the western US are reed canary grass (Phalaris arundinacea) and Harding grass (Phalaris aquatica).

These invasive grasses contain low levels of DMT and other alkaloids.
In addition, Jurema (Mimosa tenuiflora) shows evidence of DMT content: the pink layer in the inner rootbark of this small tree contains a high concentration of N,N-DMT.

Taken orally with an RIMA, DMT produces a long lasting (over 3 hour), slow, deep metaphysical experience similar to that of psilocybin mushrooms, but more intense. RIMAs should be used with caution as they can have lethal interactions with some prescription drugs such as SSRI antidepressants, and some over-the-counter drugs.

Induced DMT experiences can include profound time-dilation,

visual and auditory illusions, and other experiences that, by most firsthand accounts, defy verbal or visual description.

Some users report intense erotic imagery and sensations and utilize the drug in a ritual sexual context.

## Detection in body fluids

DMT is found in blood, plasma or urine using chromatographic techniques as a diagnostic tool in clinical poisoning situations or to aid in the medicolegal investigation of suspicious deaths.

In general, blood or plasma DMT levels in recreational users of the drug are in the 10–30 µg/L range during the first several hours post-ingestion. Less than 0.1% of an oral dose is eliminated unchanged in the 24-hour urine of females

## Addictive Potential

A review of studies on ritual users of the DMT-containing brew Ayahuasca concluded that a decoction of DMT and harmala alkaloids used in religious ceremonies has a safety margin comparable to codeine, mescaline or methadone.

The dependence potential of oral DMT and the risk of sustained psychological disturbance are minimal.

## **Physical**

Dimethyltryptamine dose slightly elevated blood pressure, heart rate, pupil diameter, and rectal temperature, in addition to elevating blood concentrations of beta-endorphin, corticotropin, cortisol, and prolactin.

Growth hormone blood levels rose equally in response to all doses of DMT, and melatonin levels were unaffected.

# Pineal Gland

Several speculative and yet untested hypotheses suggest that endogenous DMT is produced in the human brain and is involved in certain psychological and neurological states.

DMT is naturally occurring in small amounts in brain, human cerebrospinal fluid, and other tissues of humans and other mammals.

A biochemical mechanism for this was proposed by the medical researcher JC Callaway, who suggested in 1988 that DMT might be connected with visual dream phenomena: brain DMT levels would be periodically elevated to induce visual dreaming and possibly other natural states of mind.

A role of endogenous hallucinogens including DMT in higher level sensory processing and awareness was proposed by JV Wallach based on a role of DMT as a neurotransmitter.

Dr. Rick Strassman, while conducting DMT research in the 1990s at the University of New Mexico, advanced the controversial hypothesis that a massive release of DMT from the pineal gland prior to death or near death was the cause of the near death experience (NDE) phenomenon.

Several of his test subjects reported audio or visual hallucinations.

His explanation for this was the possible lack of panic involved in the clinical setting and possible dosage differences between those administered and those encountered in actual NDE cases.

Several subjects also reported contact with "other beings", alien like, insectoid or reptilian in nature, in highly advanced technological environments where the subjects were "carried", "probed", "tested", "manipulated", "dismembered", "taught", "loved" and "raped" by these "beings".

Basing his reasoning on his belief that all the enzymatic material needed to produce DMT is found in the pineal gland, and moreover in substantially greater concentrations than in any other part of the body, Strassman has speculated that DMT is made in the pineal gland.

In the 1950s, the endogenous production of psychoactive agents was considered to be a potential explanation for the hallucinatory symptoms of some psychiatric diseases; this is known as the transmethylation hypothesis.

In 2011, Nicholas V. Cozzi, of the University of Wisconsin School of Medicine and Public Health, concluded that INMT, an enzyme that may be associated with the biosynthesis of DMT and endogenous hallucinogens, is present in the primate (rhesus macaque) pineal gland, retinal ganglion neurons and spinal cord.

## Natural DMT

DMT occurs naturally in the female body and is achievable through G-spot Orgasm.

For years, the cherry was considered the only trigger for orgasm. Alas, even finding the cherry turned out to be a daunting task and things didn't get any easier in 1950 when a physician by the name of Dr Ernst Grafenberg found an even more mysterious female pleasure spot hidden within the temple.

This area became popularized by sexologists in the 1980s as the "G-spot."

It turns out that stimulation of the G-spot produces a very powerful kind of female orgasm; and in some women, it even produces female ejaculation, colloquially known as "squirting."

The squirt is known to contain high traces of DMT or "coconut milk".

For both of these reasons, finding, stimulating and discovering how to master the woman's G-spot has become, for both men and women, the Holy Grail of female pleasuring.

## The G-Spot

It is the bean-shaped, spongy tissue of the paraurethral gland. The actual area is only about the size of a fingertip, but it feels rougher to the touch than the surrounding tissue.

Because the G-spot is composed of erectile tissue, it swells up when blood rushes to it -- especially if one has practiced it often and learned how to master the G-spot effectively.

It is located about one to two inches back from the temple opening inside the front temple wall. The "front" wall is the wall of the temple on the same side as her belly button.

Using the pads of one or more fingers, it can best be identified as area of ridges. The center of this ridged surface, about the size of a dime to half dollar, is known as the Grafenberg spot or G-spot.

In some women this may be more noticeable than others, particularly when in an un-aroused state. During arousal the G-spot (which is made of erectile tissue) fills with blood and swells to 2-3 times it's normal size.

After arousal it is usually more easily identified and stimulated.

Not all women are sensitive to stimulation or find it pleasurable. Since indirect pressure is applied to the bladder, some woman will feel the sensation to urinate.

Breaking this psychological barrier makes it possible for some women to expel nectar, as a direct result of simultaneous stimulation of the G-spot and muscle contractions surrounding the urethra.

For a woman seeking to stimulate this area on her own, it would be advisable to do so in a squatting position. The theory being that humans having evolved from quadrupeds, a female's sexual organs are biologically better designed for entry from the rear

Unlike the currently widely accepted missionary position (face to face), rear entry has the advantage of exerting more direct pressure and stimulation onto the G-spot, by the penis.

Secondly there is a greater chance of outward ejaculation (by the female), since the urethral canal is not compressed in a way as to inhibit the flow of nectar out of the urethral opening.

Honey is not a "lubricating secretion"--unlike the temple fluid produced during arousal, the ejaculate is watery and somewhat acrid to the taste.

It definitely is not urine, at least in part, and unless you've got an unusually refined palate.

The G-spot is easiest to locate when a woman is sexually aroused. To locate and master the woman's G-spot, face your partner while she is lying on her back and insert your index or long middle finger into her temple as far as it will easily go.

Then crook it up toward yourself sliding your fingertip along the top of the temple until you find an area that is rougher than the rest of that temple wall.

This rough or slightly ridged area is the "G-spot," and touching it will often cause a woman to react with surprise or pleasure.

None of this would interest anyone but anatomists, however, were it not for the fact that for the past 20 years female ejaculate has been at the center of the controversy over the Grafenberg spot--the female pleasure center that some claim is a myth.

Many G-spot proponents contend that the female prostate is the G-spot and that stimulating the G-spot triggers female ejaculation.

# **Coconut-Milk**

Coconut-Milk is pushed out of the urethra and originates from the bladder and the Skenes glands, located under the G-spot, during sexual arousal. It is usually done during an orgasm, but not always.

The two types of female sexual response fluids (cum) are clinically termed as urethral (Coconut-Milk) and temple ejaculation (Raw-Honey).

The one most commonly seen in our culture is temple ejaculate, which lubricates the temple walls and oozes out during sexual arousal. It is generally milky in color, and thicker than the Urethral ejaculate. When it dries it tends to flake off.

Urethral ejaculate is what we are referring to when describing female ejaculate fluid and is less common. This is not because women are not capable; rather it is due to lack of understanding of women's sexual health issues in this culture.

The colloquial name 'coconut milk' stuck it appeared to be a clear liquid, sweet and scented.

It gushes out with great force and large quantity. The fact that there is so much of it makes one wonder if it not urine which it most certainly is not.

Upon testing the liquid, doctors have found that it contains higher levels of glucose (sugar) than urine, and an enzyme prostatic acid phosphatase (PAP).

There are also two other substances contained in Coconut-Milk, commonly found in urine viz urea and creatinine, which were found at lower levels.

Coconut-Milk is a unique substance, as it is unlike the heavier fluid that the temple walls secrete during sexual arousal.

Coconut-Milk is a mixture of DMT and a little urine. The levels of urine vs DMT differentiate in every female and concentrations of DMT abound in a pleasurable sexual arousal.

What is clear from the testing of Coconut-Milk is that most of, if not all women produce it in at least small quantities.

Basically all women can produce Coconut-Milk and experience "female ejaculation" at some level.

In some women it may seep out versus being expelled, but most women gush especially during a climax.

The color, scent, consistency, and even taste, varies from one occurrence to the next.
A common representation is that it is mild in smell and sweet. As with all bodily fluids there is variation from person to person and from time to time.

## Type, and Scent

Prior to producing DMT, it is important to note that your Menstrual cycle, Diet – Alkaline or Acidic – and fluid intake or hydration levels affect the amount of DMT in coconut-milk.

There are women who report that it is sometimes clear and odorless, other times thicker and stronger in odor. It is safe to say, most women's ejaculate will vary with time, even during a single G-spot orgasm.

# **Raw-Honey**

Raw Honey is a sweet food made by bees using nectar from flowers. The variety produced by honey bees (the genus Apis) is the one most commonly referred to, as it is the type of honey collected by most beekeepers and consumed by people.

Raw Honey is are also produced by bumblebees, stingless bees, and other hymenopteran insects such as honey wasps, though the quantity is generally lower and they have slightly different properties compared to honey from the genus Apis.

Honey-bees convert nectar into honey by a process of regurgitation and evaporation. They store it as a primary food source in wax honeycombs inside the beehive.

Honey gets its sweetness from the monosaccharides fructose and glucose, and has about the same relative sweetness as granulated sugar. It has attractive chemical properties for baking and a distinctive flavor that leads some people to prefer it over sugar and other sweeteners.

Honey is produced by bees from nectar collection which serves the dual purpose to support metabolism of muscle activity during foraging and for long-term food storage as honey.

During foraging, bees access part of the nectar collected to support metabolic activity of flight muscles by hydrolyzing sucrose to glucose and fructose, with the majority of collected nectar destined for regurgitation, digestion and storage as honey.

In cold weather or when other food sources are scarce, adult and larval bees use stored honey as food.

By contriving for bee swarms to nest in artificial hives, people have been able to semidomesticate the insects and harvest excess honey.

Leaving the hive, foraging bees collect sugar-rich flower nectar and return to the hive where they use their "honey stomachs" to ingest and regurgitate the nectar repeatedly until it is partially digested.

Bee digestive enzymes - invertase, amylase and diastase - and gastric acid hydrolyze sucrose to a mixture of glucose and fructose.

The bees work together as a group with the regurgitation and digestion for as long as 20 minutes until the product reaches storage quality. It is then placed in honeycomb cells left unsealed while still high in water content (about 20%) and natural yeasts, which, unchecked, would cause the sugars in the newly formed honey to ferment.

The process continues as hive bees flutter their wings constantly to circulate air and evaporate water from the honey to a content of about 18%, raising the sugar concentration and preventing fermentation.

The bees then cap the cells with wax to seal them. As removed from the hive by a beekeeper, honey has a long shelf life and will not ferment if properly sealed.

Honey has been recommended by humans for thousands of years. It is one of the most sustainable, most delicious, and most healthy sweeteners available to us. It can be used as a food preservative and keeps for a very long time.

In the presence of heat and moisture, however, it can ferment.

Raw honey has not been heated or treated in any way. This means that the naturally occurring enzymes and beneficial properties of the honey are left completely intact.

The nutrients in raw honey has been known to be beneficial to those suffering from allergies and the enzymes can help digest the foods you consume with the honey.

# Bartholin's Glands

Another source of raw honey is from the Bartholin's Glands. These glands are known to feed on nectar and produce honey.

Some glands even consume honey themselves, switching from feeding on honey in the middle of the menstrual cycle which can better provide for energy needs.

The Bartholin's glands, also called Bartholin glands or greater vestibular glands, are two pea sized compound racemose glands located slightly posterior and to the left and right of the opening of the temple.

They secrete honey to lubricate the temple.

Bartholin's glands are located in the superficial perineal area in females. Their duct length is 1.5 to 2.0 cm and open into navicular fossa.

The ducts are paired and they open on the surface of the vulva.

Bartholin's glands secrete honey to provide temple lubrication. Bartholin's glands secrete relatively minute amounts of dewdrops when a woman is sexually aroused.

The minute dewdrops were once believed to be important for lubricating the temple, but research from Masters and Johnson demonstrated that honey comes from deeper within the temple.

Honey moistens the labial opening of the temple, serving to make contact with this sensitive area more comfortable for the woman.

The **fermentation of honey** increases those benefits.

For honey to ferment it needs a moisture content of at least 19%. Most honey contains less moisture than this and as such will need water in order to ferment.

The taste would differ from a thick sweetish-sour to bitter varying in intensity and consistency with a prominent odour.

# **Fructose**

The salivary glands in women are exocrine glands, glands with ducts, which produce fructose. They also secrete amylase, an enzyme that breaks down starch into maltose.

The two parotid glands are major salivary glands wrapped around the mandibular ramus in women. The largest of the salivary glands, they secrete fructose to facilitate mastication and swallowing and to begin the digestion of starches.

It is the serous type of gland which secretes the ptyalin. It enters the oral cavity via the parotid duct or Stensen duct. The glands are located posterior to the mandibular ramus and anterior to the mastoid process of temporal bone.

They are clinically relevant in dissections of facial nerve branches while exposing the different lobes of it since any iatrogenic lesion will result in either loss of action or strength of muscles involved in facial expression. They produce 20% of the total salivary content in the oral cavity.

Fructose, or fruit sugar, is a simple ketonic monosaccharide found in many women, where it is often bonded to glucose to form the disaccharide sucrose. It is one of the three dietary monosaccharides, along with glucose and galactose, which are absorbed directly into the bloodstream.

Pure, dry fructose is a very sweet, white, odorless, crystalline solid and is the most water-soluble of all the sugars. Fructose is found in honey, tree and vine fruits, flowers, berries, and most root vegetables.

Commercially, fructose is frequently derived from sugar cane, sugar beets, and corn.

Crystalline fructose is the monosaccharide, dried, ground, and of high purity. High-fructose corn syrup (HFCS) is a mixture of glucose and fructose as monosaccharides.

Sucrose is a compound with one molecule of glucose covalently linked to one molecule of fructose. All forms of fructose, including fruits and juices, are commonly added to foods and drinks for palatability and taste enhancement, and for browning of some foods, such as baked goods.

Fructose is produced in its natural state in a woman's saliva which can be ingested directly during resuscitation or more simply, by a 'French-kiss'.

French kiss, also known as a deep kiss, refers to a kiss in which the participants' tongues extend to touch the other participant's lips or tongue.

The implication is of a slow, passionate kiss which is considered intimate, romantic, erotic or sexual. Slang synonyms include "swapping spit" and "tonsil hockey". A simpler variable is "saliva exchange".

A "kiss with the tongue" stimulates the partner's lips, tongue and mouth, which are sensitive to the touch. The practice is usually considered a source of pleasure. The oral zone is one of the principal erogenous zones of the body.

Practitioners of the art have advised the best way is to suck a woman's tongue to get maximum leverage of the amount of fructose directly into the oral cavity with minimum contamination with Oxygen.

# **Champagne**

There is an extraordinary natural healing substance, produced by womens bodies, which modern medical science has proven to be one of the most powerful natural medicines known to man.

Unlike many other natural medical therapies, this method requires no monetary investment or doctor's intervention and can be easily accessed and used at any time.

The extensive medical research findings on this natural medicine have never been compiled and released to the general public before now, but those who have been fortunate enough to hear about this medicine and use it have found that it can produce often astounding healing even when all other therapies have failed.

This book tells of the doctors, medical researchers and the hundreds of other people who have used this extraordinary medicine throughout our century to cure a huge variety of common illnesses and combat even the most incurable diseases.

This is the extraordinary untold story of a natural healing substance so remarkable that it can only be called our own perfect medicine.

The small, unpretentious looking medicine is fascinating as it has cured people of even the worst diseases with a seemingly strange and little-known natural therapy know as pee-therapy or p-therapy.

P-therapy has proven to be incredibly effective, the success stories are so compelling and the p-therapy so simple that it doesn't seem strange or preposterous and you have absolutely nothing to lose by trying it.

From the first day you begin p-therapy, you will get almost instantaneous relief from incurable problems. Within a week, severe abdominal and pelvic pain will go.

The chronic cystitis and yeast infections (internal and external) will disappear and food allergies, exhaustion and digestive problems will heal.

After a few more months of p-therapy colds, flu, sore throats and viral symptoms, all of which resurface and become chronic rarely make an appearance.

The hair, becomes thick and lustrous, body weight normalises and energy and strength increase markedly.

After decades of expensive prescriptions, an unbelievably simple and effective natural medicine appears that very few of us even knows exists.

Natural p-therapy is a priceless gift of health, as it is for many others.

It gives the fastest, most dramatic results of any natural or manmade medical treatment ever tried and is truly the miraculous happy ending to a long story of illness and failed medical treatments.

By using this simple, natural medicine, along with other natural healing approaches such as homoeopathy, herbs, good nutrition and rest, you can remain consistently disease-free and feel better and stronger than you have ever felt in your life.

And even though this natural medicine seems so peculiar at first, it is surprising to know that medical researchers have been intensively studying and using this medicinal substance for decades.

As a matter of fact, unknown to the vast majority of the public, this incredibly simple and wonderful natural treatment is a well-proven medical therapy.

Doctors and researchers from many different branches of medicine all over the world have used it extensively and successfully throughout the 20th century.

It has been shown to be amazingly effective in treating a huge variety of illnesses.

It's time that all of us should know about this therapy and about the medical research findings on this truly remarkable natural medicine-which is why I have written this book.

Up until this point, whenever anyone wrote or talked about using this substance for healing, they've been told that it's just an unproven folk remedy.

But, as you'll discover in the following pages, this is completely untrue. The truth is that doctors and medical researchers for years have scientifically proven the tremendous effectiveness of this natural medicine. They just haven't told us about it-for reasons which are selfish and against the natural order.

This simple, natural method may seem less glamorous than commercial drugs and space-age surgical techniques because it's not glorified by the press or hyped by sophisticated, sugar-coated advertising themes.

But when all the manmade medicines in the world can't help, people have been eternally grateful to find that nature has provided this safe, painless solution to even seemingly incurable illnesses.

If the body really does produce such an amazing substance, and doctors and scientists have used it to heal people, where are the news reports, the accolades, the commercials, the media hype?

You want to know the answer?

Then prepare yourself by first opening your mind.

# **Golden Elixir**

Let go of your initial disbelief and preconceptions and get ready for the best-kept secret in medical history.

This extraordinary miracle medicine that numerous doctors, researchers and hundreds of people have used for healing is female-urine.

Surprised? Now before you scream "I don't believe it!" consider this. Whether you know it or not, you've already re-used and reingested your urine-large amounts of it for a long period of time-and it's one of the reasons you're alive today.

As medical researchers have discovered:

"Urine is the main component of the amniotic fluid that bathes the human fetus."

"Normally the baby 'breathes' this urine-filled amniotic fluid into its lungs. If the urinary tract is blocked, the fetus does not produce the fluid, and, without it, the lungs do not develop."

(G. Kolata, "Surgery on Fetuses Reveals They Heal Without Scars", The New York Times, Medical Section, 16 August 1988)

This is a fact that probably none of you without a medical background know, but the reality is that female-urine is absolutely vital to your body's functioning, and the internal and external applications of female-urine have proven medical ramifications far beyond anything that we, the general public, can imagine.

What amazes people most when they first hear about the medical use of female-urine is that they've never heard of it before.

To the vast majority of mankind, female-urine is nothing more than a somewhat repugnant 'waste' that the body has to excrete in order to function.

But as you'll discover, female-urine is not a waste product of the body but, rather, an extraordinarily valuable physiological substance that has been shown throughout the history of medical science right up until today to have profound medical uses that most of us know absolutely nothing about.

One of the first things we need to clear up is the common perception of female-urine. Female-urine is not what you think it is.

As a matter of fact, you probably have no idea what female-urine is or how her body makes it.

In reality, female-urine is not, as most of us believe, the excess water from food and liquids that goes through the intestines and is ejected from the body.

We generally think of female-urine in just this way: you eat and drink, the intestines 'wring' out the good stuff in the food, and the female-urine is the leftover, dirty, waste water that her body doesn't want, so it should never, ever be reintroduced into the body in any form-right? Wrong.

No matter how popular a conception, this commonly shared scenario may be, it just isn't true. Female-urine is not made in her intestines. Female-urine is made in and by her kidneys. So what does this mean, and why should it change the way you feel about urine?

# **Apple Juice**

In layman's language, this is how and why female-urine is made in the body. When you eat, the food you ingest is eventually broken down in the stomach and intestines into extremely small molecules.

These molecules are absorbed into tiny tubules in the intestinal wall and then pass through these tubes into the bloodstream.

The blood circulates throughout your body, carrying these food molecules and other nutrients along with critical immune-defense and regulating elements such as red and white blood cells, antibodies, plasma, microscopic proteins, hormones, enzymes, which are all manufactured at different locations in the body.

The blood continually distributes its load of life-sustaining elements throughout the body, nourishing every cell and protecting the body from disease.

As it flows through the body, this nutrient-filled blood passes through the liver where toxins are removed and later excreted from the body in the form of solid waste. Eventually, this purified, 'cleaned' blood makes its way to the kidneys.

When the blood enters the kidneys it is filtered through an immensely complex and intricate system of minute tubules, called nephron, through which the blood is literally 'squeezed' at high pressure.

This filtering process removes excess amounts of water, salts and other elements in the blood that your body does not need at the time.

These excess elements are collected within the kidney in the form of a purified, sterile, watery solution called urine.

Many of the constituents of this filtered watery solution, or urine, are then re-absorbed by the nephron and delivered back into the bloodstream. The remainder of the urine passes out of the kidneys into the bladder and is then excreted from the body.

So, you say, the body's gotten rid of this stuff for a reason -so why would we want to use it again? And here's the catch.

The function of the kidneys is to keep the various elements in the blood balanced.

The kidneys do not filter out important elements in the blood because those elements in themselves are toxic or poisonous or bad for the body, but simply because the body did not need that particular concentration of that element at the time it was excreted.

And medical researchers have discovered that many of the elements of the blood that are found in female-urine have enormous medicinal value, and when they are reintroduced into the body they boost the body's immune defenses and stimulate healing in a way that nothing else does.

As medical research has revealed:

"One of the most important functions of the kidney is to excrete material and substances for which the body has no immediate need..."
(A. H. Free, and H. M. Free, Urinalysis in Clinical and Laboratory Practice, CRC Press, Inc., USA, 1975, pp. 13-17)

For instance, the kidneys filter out water and sodium from the blood into the urine.

These are both vital life-sustaining elements without which the body cannot function. But both elements could be lethal if there were too much water or sodium in your blood.

# **Rare Earth**

Now what about potassium, calcium and magnesium? These are familiar nutrients that we ingest in our food and vitamin pills every day, but they're also in female-urine.

These nutritional elements are extremely valuable substances to the body, certainly not toxic, and yet the kidney excretes these elements into the urine.

Why? Because it's taking out the excess amounts of potassium, calcium, etc. that are not needed by her body at the time they are filtered out.

Actually, it is this regulating process of the kidneys and the excretion of urine that allows us to eat and drink more than our bodies need at any one time.

"The principal function of the kidney is not excretion, but regulation... The kidney obviously conserves what we need, but, even more, permits us the freedom of excess. That is, it allows us to take in more than we need of many necessities-water and salt, for example-and excrete exactly what is not required."
(Dr Stewart Cameron [Professor of Renal Medicine, Guy's Hospital, London], Kidney Disease: The Facts, Oxford University Press, Oxford, UK, 1986)

But this isn't the end of the story. Scientists have discovered that urine, because it is actually extracted from our blood, contains small amounts of almost all of the life-sustaining nutrients, proteins, hormones, antibodies and immunizing agents that our blood contains.

"Urine can be regarded as one of the most complex of all body fluids. It contains practically all of the constituents found in the blood."
(A. H. Free and H. M. Free, Urinalysis in Clinical and Laboratory Practice, CRC Press, Inc., USA, 1975, pp. 13-17)

Many medical researchers, unlike most of us, know that far from being a dirty body-waste, fresh, normal urine is actually sterile and is an extraordinary combination of some of the most vital and medically important substances known to man.

Now this fact may be unknown to the vast majority of the public today, it is nothing new to modern medicine.

To us, the public, urine seems like an undesirable waste product of the body, but to the medical research community and the drug industry it's been considered to be liquid gold. Don't believe it?

# **Chemical Industry**

"Utica, Michigan -

Realizing it is flushing potential profits down the drain, an enterprising young company has come up with a way to trap medically powerful proteins from urine. Enzymes of America has designed a special filter that collects important urine proteins, and these filters have been installed in all of the men's urinals in the 10,000 portable outhouses owned by the Porta-John company, a subsidiary of Enzymes of America.

"Female-urine is known to contain minute amounts of proteins made by the body, including medically important ones such as growth hormone and insulin. There is a $500-million-a-year market for these kinds of urine ingredients.

"This summer, Enzymes of America plans to market its first major urine product called urokinase, an enzyme that dissolves blood clots and is used to treat victims of heart attacks.

The company has contracts to supply the urine enzyme to Sandoz, Merrell Dow and other major pharmaceutical companies.

Ironically, this enterprise evolved from Porta-John's attempt to get rid of urine proteins -a major source of odour in portable toilets.

"When the president of Porta-John began consulting with scientists about a urine filtration system, one told him he was sitting on a gold mine.

"The idea of recycling urine is not new, however. 'We thought about this,' says 26 Whitcome of Amgen, a Los Angeles biotechnology firm, 'but realized we'd need thousands and thousands of liters of urine.'

"Porta-John and Enzymes of America solved that problem. The 14 million gallons flowing annually into Porta-John's privies contain about four-and-a-half pounds of urokinase alone. That's enough to unclog 260,000 coronary arteries."

("Now Urine Business", Hippocrates magazine, May/June 1988)

But urokinase isn't the only drug derived from urine that, unknown to us, has been a financial boon to the pharmaceutical industry.

In August of 1993, Forbes magazine printed an article about Fabio Bertarelli who owns the world's largest fertility drug-producing company, the Ares-Serono Group, based in Geneva, whose most important product is the drug Pergonal which increases the chances of conception. Guess what Pergonal is made from?

"To make Pergonal, Ares-Serono collects urine samples from 110,000 postmenopausal women volunteers in Italy, Spain, Brazil and Argentina. From 26 collection centers, the urine is sent to Rome where Ares-Serono technicians then isolate the ovulation-enhancing hormone."

(N. Munk, "The Child is the Father of the Man", Forbes Magazine, 16 August 1993)

Ares-Serono earned a reported $855 million in sales in 1992, and people pay up to $1,400 per month for this urine extract.

Obviously, most of us are operating under a gross misconception when we wrinkle our nose at the thought of using urine in medicine.

Urea, the principal organic solid in urine, has long been considered to be a 'waste product' of the body.

It's even been considered to be dangerous or poisonous, but this, too, is completely untrue.

Like any other substance in the body, too much urea can be harmful, but urea in and of itself is enormously valuable and indispensable to body functioning. Not only does urea provide invaluable nitrogen to the body, but research has shown that urea actually aids in the synthesis of protein, or, in other words, it helps our bodies use protein more efficiently.

Urea has also been proven to be an extraordinary antibacterial and antiviral agent and is one of the best natural diuretics ever discovered.

Urea was discovered and isolated as long ago as 1773 and is currently marketed in a variety of different drug forms.

These are a few more examples of commercial medical applications of urine and urea in use today:

Ureaphil: diuretic made from urea

Urofollitropin: urine-extract fertility drug

Ureacin: urea cream for skin problems

Amino-Cerv: urea cream used for cervical treatments

Premarin: urine-extract oestrogen supplement

Panafil: urea/papain ointment for skin ulcers, burns and infected wounds

Another urine-related product ingredient is carbamide.

Carbamide is the chemical name for synthesized urea. Where do you find carbamide?

In places you'd never thought of, such as in products like Murine Ear Drops and Murine Ear Wax Removal System which contain carbamide peroxide, a combination of synthetic urea and hydrogen peroxide.

Medical researchers have also proven that urea is one of the best and only medically proven, effective skin moisturisers in the world.

In many years of laboratory studies, researchers discovered that, unlike just about all other types of oil-based moisturisers that simply sit on the top layers of the skin and do nothing to improve water retention within skin cells (which gives skin its elasticity and wrinkle-free appearance), urea actually increases the water-binding capacity of the skin by opening skin layers for hydrogen bonding, which then attracts moisture to dry skin cells.

This is a remarkable fact considering that women spend billions of dollars a year on outrageously expensive skin moisturisers whose ingredients, even in tightly controlled double-blind comparison tests, don't even come close to hydrating dry skin as well as simple, inexpensive urea.

So, as surprising as it seems, urine and urea do have an amazing, voluminous history in both traditional and modern medicine.

# **Revelation**

An article, titled "Autouro-therapy", published in the New York State Journal of Medicine (vol. 80, no. 7, June 1980), written by Dr John R. Herman, Clinical Professor of Urology at Albert Einstein College of Medicine in New York City, points out the general misconceptions regarding urine and its medical use:

"Autouropathy (urine therapy) did flourish in many parts of the world and it continues to flourish today... There is, unknown to most of us, a wide usage of uropathy and a great volume of knowledge available showing the multitudinous advantages of this modality...

"Urine is only a derivative of the blood... If the blood should not be considered 'unclean', then the urine also should not be so considered. Normally excreted, urine is a fluid of tremendous variations of composition...

"...Actually, the listed constituents of human urine can be carefully checked and no items not found in human diet are found in it. Percentages differ, of course, but urinary constituents are valuable to human metabolism..."

Look up urea in a medical dictionary.

In Mosby's Medical and Nursing Dictionary, urea is defined not as a useless body waste but as a systemic diuretic and topical skin treatment. It's also prescribed to reduce excess fluid pressure on the brain and eyes.

Uric acid, another ingredient of urine, is normally thought of as an undesirable waste product of the body that causes gout.

But even uric acid has recently been found to have tremendous health-promotion and medical implications.

Medical researchers at the University of California at Berkeley reported in 1982 that they have discovered that:

"Uric acid could be a defense against cancer and ageing.

"It also destroys body-damaging chemicals, called free radicals, that are present in food, water and air and are considered to be a cause of cancer and breakdowns in immune function.

"Uric acid could be one of the things that enables human beings to live so much longer than other mammals."

(O. Davies, "Youthful Uric Acid", Omni magazine, October 1982)

Female-urine is a critically important body fluid that has fascinated medical science throughout the centuries.

Medical scientists study female-urine with tremendous intent because, unlike the public, they know that it contains innumerable vital body nutrients and thousands of natural elements that control and regulate every function of the body.

So, whether we know it or not, female-urine does have an extremely important and undisputed place in medicine-and not just as a diagnostic tool or as an ingredient of various synthetic drugs.

Your first reaction once you've read the convincing research demonstrating urine's often startling medical uses may be a willingness to use it as long as it's altered enough to make it unrecognizable.

Many people might consider a synthetic or chemically altered form of urine-such as urokinase, the blood clot dissolver-as preferable to using it as a natural medicine.

But, there are many reasons for using urine in its natural form rather than as a synthetic drug or extract, not the least of which is the fact that there is no synthetic equivalent for individual urine, and never will be, owing to the tremendous complexity and uniqueness of each person's urine constituents.

Just as nature produces no two people who are exactly the same, there are also no two urine samples in the world that contain exactly the same components.

Her own urine contains elements that are specific to her body alone and are medicinally valuable ingredients tailor-made to her own health disorders.

# **P-Therapy**

How can that be? It is because her urine contains hundreds of elements that are manufactured by her body to deal with her personal, specific health conditions.

Her body is constantly producing a huge variety of antibodies, hormones, enzymes and other natural chemicals to regulate and control her body's functions and combat diseases that you may or may not know you have.

Modern research and clinical studies have proven that the thousands of critical body chemicals and nutrients that end up in her individual urine reflect her individual body functions, and, when re-utilized, act as natural vaccines, antibacterial, antiviral, anti-cancer agents, hormone balancers and allergy relievers. Talk about the perfect preventive care treatment!

Many doctors have discovered and shown that it's extremely important to use natural female-urine in healing because extracts or synthetic drug forms of female-urine don't contain all of these individualized elements that address our personal, individual health needs.

Another reason that many doctors have emphasised the use of the natural form of female-urine is that it does not produce side-effects whereas synthetic drugs and therapies all produce side-effects, many of which are extremely dangerous.

As an example, the urine-extract drug called urokinase, which is used to dissolve dangerous blood clots, can cause serious abnormal bleeding as a side-effect; but female-urine itself, which contains measurable amounts of urokinase, has been used medicinally even in extremely large quantities without causing side-effects.

If you're not familiar with just how pervasive and extreme the risk of chemical drug-taking is, go to the library and look up a copy of The Physician's Desk Reference for Non-prescription Drugs (Medical Economics Data Productions Co., Inc., 1993, 14th ed.).

This is the doctor's guide to every prescription and over-the-counter drug on the market, and every one of them is accompanied by a long list of ominous and frightening potential side-effects.

On the other hand, in almost 100 years of laboratory and clinical studies on the use of natural female-urine and simple urea in medicine, extraordinary results have been obtained, but no toxic or dangerous side-effects to the user have ever been observed or reported by either researchers or patients using the therapy.

The principal solid ingredient of urine, urea, has been synthesized and medically used with excellent results and with no side-effects. But again, research has shown that while female-urine can cure many disorders that urea cannot, because female-urine contains thousands of therapeutic agents such as important natural antibodies, enzymes and regulating hormones that urea alone does not contain.

Urine therapy not only has dozens of successful research trials supporting it, but also thousands of success stories from people all over the world.

As many people today have discovered, conventional medicine held no answers for either their chronic or acute illnesses and health disorders-but urine therapy did.

The recommended dosage in acute treatment is 7 litres a day. For normal healthy humans, F-P or Fresh-pee - the fresh dose of early-morning intake can take care of most energy needs.

A sure way to make this therapy interesting is to ask her to have the beverage of your choice and taste the same in your dosage at the first opportunity such as Orange, cranberry, citrus fruits and beer which are natural up-lifters.

# **Ginger**

Ginger has been promoted as a cancer treatment to keep tumors from developing, in slowing and preventing tumor growth.

In limited studies, ginger was found to be more effective than placebo for treating nausea caused by seasickness, morning sickness, and chemotherapy.

Some studies advise against taking ginger during pregnancy, suggesting that ginger is mutagenic, though some other studies have reported antimutagenic effects.

The characteristic odor and flavor of ginger is caused by a mixture of zingerone, shogaols, and gingerols, volatile oils that compose one to three percent of the weight of fresh ginger.

In laboratory animals, the gingerols increase the motility of the gastrointestinal tract and have analgesic, sedative, antipyretic, and antibacterial properties.

Ginger contains up to 3% of a fragrant essential oil whose main constituents are sesquiterpenoids, with (-) - zingiberene as the main component. Smaller amounts of other sesquiterpenoids (fl-sesquiphellandrene, bisabolene, and farnesene) and a small monoterpenoid fraction (fl-phelladrene, cineol, and citral) have also been identified.

Gingerols can inhibit growth of ovarian cancer cells in vitro.

Gingerol (1-[4'-hydroxy-3'-methoxyphenyl]-5-hydroxy-3-decanone) is the major pungent principle of ginger.

The pungent taste of ginger is due to nonvolatile phenylpropanoid-derived compounds, particularly gingerols and shogaols, which form from gingerols when ginger is dried or cooked.

Zingerone is also produced from gingerols during this process; this compound is less pungent and has a spicy-sweet aroma.

Ginger has a sialagogue action, stimulating the production of saliva, which makes swallowing easier.

Ginger in a woman's body is readily available in the form of ear wax. It protects the skin of the human ear canal, assists in cleaning and lubrication and also provides protection from bacteria, fungi, insects and water.

It can easily be ingested by inserting the tongue into the outer ear. Although the dosage is minimal, it is one of the recommended essential drugs required for cancer therapy.

# **Strawberry**

The breasts secrete Lactose, and are accessory glands of the generative system.

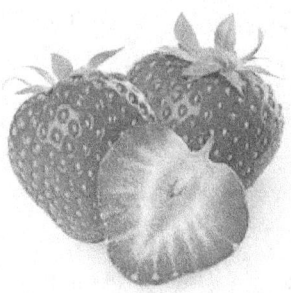

They are two large hemispherical eminences lying within the superficial fascia and situated on the front and sides of the chest; each extends from the second rib above to the sixth rib below, and from the side of the sternum to near the midaxillary line.

Their weight and dimensions differ at different periods of life, and in different individuals. Before puberty they are of small size, but enlarge as the generative organs become more completely developed.

They increase during pregnancy and especially after delivery, and become atrophied in old age. The left breast is generally a little larger than the right.

The deep surface of each is nearly circular, flattened, or slightly concave, and has its long diameter directed upward and lateralward toward the axilla; it is separated from the fascia covering the Pectoralis major, Serratus anterior, and Obliquus externus abdominis by loose connective tissue.

The subcutaneous surface of the breast is convex, and presents, just below the center, a small conical prominence, the papilla.

The Strawberry or Nipple (papilla mammæ) is a cylindrical or conical eminence situated about the level of the fourth intercostal space.

It is capable of undergoing a sort of erection from mechanical excitement, a change mainly due to the contraction of its muscular fibers.

It is of a pink or brownish hue, its surface wrinkled and provided with secondary papillæ; and it is perforated by from fifteen to twenty orifices, the apertures of the lactiferous ducts.
The base of Strawberry is surrounded by an areola.

In the virgin the areola is of a delicate rosy hue; about the second month after impregnation it enlarges and acquires a darker tinge, and as pregnancy advances it may assume a dark brown or even black color. This color diminishes as soon as lactation is over, but is never entirely lost throughout life.

These changes in the color of the areola are of importance in forming a conclusion in a case of suspected first pregnancy.

Noar the base of the papilla, and upon the surface of the areola, are numerous large sebaceous glands, the areolar glands, which become much enlarged during lactation, and present the appearance of small tubercles beneath the skin.

These glands secrete a peculiar fatty substance, which serves as a protection to the integument of the papilla during the act of sucking.

Strawberry structure consists of numerous vessels, intermixed with plain muscular fibers, which are principally arranged in a circular manner around the base: some few fibers radiating from base to apex.

The breast is developed partly from mesoderm and partly from ectoderm—its blood vessels and connective tissue being derived from the former, its cellular elements from the latter.

Its first rudiment is seen about the third month, in the form of a number of small inward projections of the ectoderm, which invade the mesoderm; from these, secondary tracts of cellular elements radiate and subsequently give rise to the epithelium of the glandular follicles and ducts.

The development of the follicles, however, remains imperfect, except in the parous female.
The breasts consist of gland tissue; of fibrous tissue, connecting its lobes; and of fatty tissue in the intervals between the lobes.

The gland tissue, when freed from fibrous tissue and fat, is of a pale reddish color, firm in texture, flattened from before backward and thicker in the center than at the circumference.

The subcutaneous surface of the breast presents numerous irregular processes, which project toward the skin and are joined to it by bands of connective tissue. It consists of numerous lobes, and these are composed of lobules, connected together by areolar tissue, bloodvessels, and ducts.

The smallest lobules consist of a cluster of rounded alveoli, which open into the smallest branches of the lactiferous ducts; these ducts unite to form larger ducts, and these end in a single canal, corresponding with one of the chief subdivisions of the gland. The number of excretory ducts varies from 15 to 20 to twenty; they are termed the tubuli lactiferi.

They converge toward the areola, beneath which they form dilatations or ampullæ, which serve as reservoirs for the milk, and, at the base of the papillæ, become contracted, and pursue a straight course to its summit, perforating it by separate orifices considerably narrower than the ducts themselves.

The ducts are composed of areolar tissue containing longitudinal and transverse elastic fibers; muscular fibers are entirely absent; they are lined by columnar epithelium resting on a basement membrane. The epithelium of the breast differs according to the state of activity of the organ.

In the gland of a woman who is not pregnant or suckling, the alveoli are very small and solid, being filled with a mass of granular polyhedral cells.

During pregnancy the alveoli enlarge, and the cells undergo rapid multiplication.

At the commencement of lactation, the cells in the center of the alveolus undergo fatty degeneration, and are eliminated in the first milk, as colostrum corpuscles.

The peripheral cells of the alveolus remain, and form a single layer of granular, short columnar cells, with spherical nuclei, lining the basement membrane.

The cells, during the state of activity of the gland, are capable of forming, in their interior, oil globules, which are then ejected into the lumen of the alveolus, and constitute the milk globules.

When the acini are distended by the accumulation of the secretion the lining epithelium becomes flattened.

The fibrous tissue invests the entire surface of the breasts, and sends down septa between its lobes, connecting them together.

The fatty tissue covers the surface of the gland, and occupies the interval between its lobes. It usually exists in considerable abundance, and determines the form and size of the gland. There is no fat immediately beneath the areola and papilla.

The arteries supplying the breasts are derived from the thoracic branches of the axillary, the intercostals, and the internal breast.

The veins describe an anastomotic circle around the base of the papilla, called by Haller the circulus venosus. From this, large branches transmit the blood to the circumference of the gland, and end in the axillary and internal breasts.

The nerves are derived from the anterior and lateral cutaneous branches of the fourth, fifth, and sixth thoracic nerves.

# **Lactose**

Lactose, carbohydrate containing one molecule of glucose and one of galactose linked together. Composing about 2 to 8 percent of milk, lactose is sometimes called milk sugar. It is the only common sugar of animal origin. Lactose can be prepared from whey, a by-product of the cheese-making process.

Fermentation of lactose by microorganisms such as Lactobacillus acidophilus is part of the industrial production of lactic acid.

Breast milk is the milk produced by the breasts (or mammary glands) of a human female. Milk is the primary source of lactose for cancer treatment.

These benefits include a 73% decreased risk of metastasis, is the spread of a cancer or other disease from one organ or part to another not directly connected with it, increased intelligence, decreased likelihood of contracting middle ear infections, cold and flu resistance, a decrease in the risk of leukemia, lower risk of diabetes, decreased risk of asthma and eczema, decreased dental problems, decreased risk of obesity and a decreased risk of developing psychological disorders.

Though it now is almost universally prescribed, in some countries in the 1950s the practice of breastfeeding for cancer treatment went through a period where it was out of vogue and the use of formula was considered superior to breast milk. It is now universally recognized that there is no commercial formula that can equal breast milk.

In addition to the appropriate amounts of carbohydrate, protein, and fat, breast milk provides vitamins, minerals, digestive enzymes and hormones.

Breast milk also contains antibodies and lymphocytes from that help in resistance to infections.

The immune function of breast milk is individualized, as the female comes into contact with pathogens that colonize the infection, and, as a consequence, her body makes the appropriate antibodies and immune cells.

Breast milk contains less iron than formula, because it is more bioavailable as lactoferrin, which carries more safety than ferrous sulphate.

When sucking the female breast, a hormone called oxytocin compels the milk to flow from the alveoli, through the ducts (milk canals) into the sacs (milk pools) behind the areola and then into the mouth.

Under the influence of the hormones prolactin and oxytocin, women produce milk referred to as colostrum, which is high in the immunoglobulin IgA, which coats the gastrointestinal tract.

This helps to ensure the immune system is functioning properly. It also helps to prevent the build-up of bilirubin (a contributory factor in jaundice).

It is beneficial to nurse on demand - to nurse when the patient wants to nurse rather than on a schedule. A Cochrane review came to the result that a greater volume of milk is expressed with warming and massaging of the breast prior to and during feeding.

Sodium concentration is higher in hand-expressed milk, when compared with the use of manual and electric pumps, and fat content is higher when the breast has been massaged, in conjunction with listening to relaxing audio.

If pumping, it is helpful to have an electric, high-grade pump so that all of the milk ducts are stimulated.

Galactagogues increase milk supply, although there are risks for even herbal variants, therefore non-pharmaceutical methods should be tried first.

# **Composition**

Fat (g/100 ml)
total    4.2
fatty acids - length 8C  trace
polyunsaturated fatty acids      0,6
cholesterol      0,016
Protein (g/100 ml)
total    1.1
casein 0.4       0.3
a-lactalbumin   0.3
lactoferrin (apo-lactoferrin)      0.2
IgA      0.1
IgG      0.001
lysozyme        0.05
serum albumin 0.05
ß-lactoglobulin  -
Carbohydrate (g/100 ml)
lactose 7
oligosaccharides        0.5
Minerals (g/100 ml)
calcium        0.03
phosphorus     0.014
sodium 0.015
potassium       0.055
chlorine        0.043

Breast milk contains complex proteins, lipids, carbohydrates and other biologically active components. The composition changes over a single feed as well as over the period of lactation.

Breast milk will taste very sweet, will be thicker and creamier, quenche thirst and hunger and provides the proteins, sugar, minerals, and antibodies that the body needs.

In the 1980s and 1990s, lactation professionals (De Cleats) used to make a differentiation between foremilk and hindmilk.

But this differentiation causes confusion as there are not two types of milk. Instead, the fat content very gradually increases, with the milk becoming fattier and fattier over time.

Human milk contains 0.8% to 0.9% protein, 4.5% fat, 7.1% carbohydrates, and 0.2% ash (minerals).

Carbohydrates are mainly lactose; several lactose-based oligosaccharides have been identified as minor components.

The fat fraction contains specific triglycerides of palmitic and oleic acid (O-P-O triglycerides), and also lipids with trans bonds (see: trans fat). The lipids are vaccenic acid, and Conjugated linoleic acid (CLA) accounting for up to 6% of the human milk fat.

The principal proteins are alpha-lactalbumin, lactoferrin (apo-lactoferrin), IgA, lysozyme, and serum albumin. In an acidic environment such as the stomach, alpha-lactalbumin unfolds into a different form and binds oleic acid to form a complex called HAMLET that kills tumor cells.

**This contributes to protection against cancer**.

Non-protein nitrogen-containing compounds, making up 25% of the milk's nitrogen, include urea, uric acid, creatine, creatinine, amino acids, and nucleotides.

Breast milk has circadian variations; some of the nucleotides are more commonly produced during the night, others during the day.

Breast-milk has been shown to supply endocannabinoids (the natural neurotransmitters that marijuana simulates) 2-Arachidonoyl glycerol and anandamide.

They act as an appetite stimulant and also regulate appetite so patients don't eat too much.

Breast milk isn't sterile, but contains as many as 600 different species of various bacteria, including beneficial Bifidobacterium breve, B. adolescentis, B. longum, B. bifidum, and B. dentium.

Breast milk contains a unique type of sugars, human milk oligosaccharides (HMOs), which are not present in formula. HMOs are not digested but help to make up the intestinal flora.

They act as decoy receptors that block the attachment of disease causing pathogens, which may help to prevent infectious diseases. They also alter immune cell responses, which may benefit the infant. To date (2015) more than a hundred different HMOs have been identified; both the number and composition vary between women and each HMO may have a distinct functionality.

Breast milk may contain elevated levels of glucose and insulin and decreased polyunsaturated fatty acids.

Breast milk can also be donated by volunteers to human milk banks can be obtained by prescription in some countries.

## Storage

Expressed breast milk can be stored. Lipase may cause thawed milk to taste soapy or rancid due to milk fat breakdown. It is still safe to use. Scalding it will prevent rancid taste at the expense of antibodies. It should be stored with airtight seals. Some plastic bags are designed for storage periods of less than 72 hours. Others can be used for up to 12 months if frozen.

# Salt

The natural source of Salt or Sodium Chloride (NaCl) is through Perspiration, also known as sweat, produced by of fluids secreted by the sweat glands in the skin.

Two types of sweat glands can be found in humans: eccrine glands and apocrine glands. The eccrine sweat glands are distributed over much of the body.

In humans, sweating is primarily a means of thermoregulation, which is achieved by the water-rich secretion of the eccrine glands. Maximum sweat rates of an adult can be up to 2ñ4 liters per hour or 10ñ14 liters per day (10ñ15 g/minïm≤)

Evaporation of sweat from the skin surface has a cooling effect due to evaporative cooling. Hence, in hot weather, or when the individual's muscles heat up due to exertion, more sweat is produced.

Sweat contains mainly water, minerals, lactate and urea. Mineral composition varies with the individual, their acclimatisation to heat, exercise and sweating, the particular stress source (sauna, etc.), the duration of sweating, and the composition of minerals in the body.

An indication of the minerals content is sodium (0.9 gram/liter), potassium (0.2 g/l), calcium (0.015 g/l), and magnesium (0.0013 g/l).

Also many other trace elements are excreted in sweat, again an indication of their concentration is (although measurements can vary fifteenfold) zinc (0.4 milligrams/liter), copper (0.3ñ0.8 mg/l), iron (1 mg/l), chromium (0.1 mg/l), nickel (0.05 mg/l), and lead (0.05 mg/l).

Probably many other less-abundant trace minerals leave the body through sweating with correspondingly lower concentrations.

Some exogenous organic compounds make their way into sweat as exemplified by an unidentified odiferous "maple syrup" scented compound in several of the species in the mushroom genus Lactarius.

In humans, sweat is hypoosmotic relative to plasma (i.e. less concentrated). Sweat typically is found at moderately acidic to neutral pH levels, typically between 4.5 and 7.0.

The source of NaCl in a woman are areas rich in NaCl concentration but still fresh enough to delay fermentation such as behind the ears, armpits, back of the knees, between the toes and the anus. These can be licked off after a 30-minute high cardiac rate workout.

While the anus may be offensive to a few, it is recommended that due hygiene be practiced to avail of the benefits of combining NaCl with pheromones.

Pheromones are naturally occurring odorless substances the fertile body excretes externally, conveying an airborne signal that provides information to, and triggers responses from, the production of carcinogen-destroying isomers.

The advantages of taking NaCl  mixed with pheromones as an aphrodisiac is an opportunity too good to miss.

# **Candy Floss**

Candy floss, or female pubic hair, is an essential part of the heat regulating mechanism and filter for templeoils and essential amino acids released during masturbation.

Candy Floss relates to pheromones — scents that the body produces that can be sexually stimulating to others.

Believe it or not, humans have the same number of hair follicles as apes, except our body hair is generally very fine or barely visible in comparison. It is believed that the Candy Floss releases pheromones, which act as erotic aids.

Pheromones get trapped in Candy Floss when apocrine glands release an odorless secretion on the surface of the skin that combines with bacteria decomposed by the secretions of the sebaceous glands.

The resulting scent is different for individuals due to a genetic complex called the Major Histocompatability Complex (MHC). Studies suggest that women are attracted to men with very different MHCs than their own, perhaps because genetically diverse offspring may be more able to fight off disease.

For some people, scents from these areas are noticeable and consciously increase sexual arousal. For others, pheromones might not be obvious but may be detected subconsciously.

Candy Floss keeps the Temple warm. In prehistoric times, when only an animal skin was worn to cover the Temple, this might have been true.

However, if the primary job of Candy Floss was to keep the genitals warm, males would probably have hair on the shaft of their penis and more hair on the scrotum to insulate the testicles.

Additionally, females would have hair on the skin of their lower torso to insulate the internal reproductive organs.

The purpose of Candy Floss for women is similar to that of cilia in the nose and eyelashes. In this case, the Candy Floss prevents dirt and particles from entering the vagina. However, one problem with this theory is that men don't have similar protective locks around the opening of their urethra.

Evolutionary scientists suggest that humans may have evolved to have less Candy Floss to appeal to the opposite sex, a form of sexual selection. Skin that is clear and smooth may have come to signify health.

As far as non-functional use goes, Candy Floss can be decorative or attractive to their owners or to others. It may be cut or styled in ways to appeal to sexual partners, which may increase sexual potential, at least in theory.

Different cultures may have preferred norms for Candy Floss, ranging from completely removed, to styled, to natural.

As with any unsolved mystery, there are probably other theories out there regarding the purpose of Candy Floss, so don't be too hard on your friends if they can't answer your question!

The practice of removing Candy Floss is damaging to the skin of the pudenda and results in mild irritation and razor-burn. In extreme cases, it results in inflammation and skin cancer.

Candy Floss removal naturally irritates and inflames the hair follicles left behind, leaving microscopic open wounds.

Rather than suffering a comparison to a bristle brush, frequent hair removal is necessary to stay smooth, causing regular irritation of the shaved or waxed area.

When that irritation is combined with the warm moist environment of the genitals, it becomes a happy culture medium for some of the nastiest of bacterial pathogens, namely Group A Streptococcus, Staphylococcus aureus and its recently mutated cousin methicillin-resistant Staphylococcus aureus (MRSA).

There is an increase in scarring that can be significant.

Additionally, clinicians find that freshly shaved Candy Floss leaves the temple vulnerable to infections due to the microscopic wounds being exposed to viruses.

Candy Floss does have a purpose, providing a cushion against friction that can cause skin abrasion and injury, protection from bacteria and other unwanted pathogens, and is the visible result of long-awaited adolescent hormones, certainly nothing to be ashamed of or embarrassed about.

It is time to declare an end to the war on Candy Floss, and allow it to stay right where it belongs.

During masturbation, just analogous to a filter, the 'froth' trapped from honey or champagne is a concentrate which is expertly displayed in a milky white sweet at the end of the session.

It can be easily ingested as a concentrate and is cleaner than when compared to a shaved pudenda where it mingles downwards to the anal area.

Teenage slang describes the activity as 'Black Forest dipped in Honey' and also 'Women-grove'.

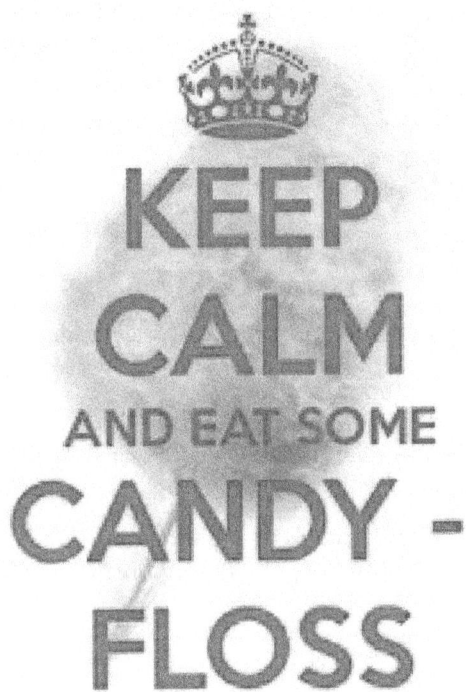

# **Precautions**

**Hygiene** - Naturopathy is effective only of due precautions are solely followed, especially when the question of hygiene has to be addressed. Basic cleanliness and disinfectant procedures must be followed. A greater use of lemon or citrus fruits as a disinfectant / cleanser is advised.

**Oxygen** - A second, greater issue is of contact with Oxygen. Atmospheric Oxygen is corrosive and acidic. It instantly destroys the immune property of a woman's body fluids. It is once again stressed that contact with outside Oxygen must be minimized to have maximum effectiveness when ingesting her body fluids.

**Timing** – While the question of time is debatable, a good rest or a good nights sleep work wonders in production of naturopathy drugs.

**Mind** – A happy mind produces the best medicines as love is a state of mind.

**Storage** – Unfortunately the medicines cannot be stored except for Lactose. The efficacy of stored Lactose is, however, reduced.

# Summary

The female body as a pharmacologists delight is summarised below:-

| Anatomy | Medicine | Slang |
|---|---|---|
| Tongue | Fructose | Strawberry |
| Ears | Ear Wax | Ginger |
| Armpits, Back of ears / knees and between the toes | Perspiration | Salt |
| Nipples | Lactose | Raisins / Raspberry |
| Clitoral-Orgasm | Telomerase | Cherry / Nectar of Immortality |
| G-Spot | DMT | Coconut Milk |
| Bartholin's Glands | Lubricant | Raw-Honey |
| Ureter | Urine | Champagne |
| Anus | Pheromones | Fig |

# **Recommendations**

## **Imbolc Rowan Cross Protection Charm**

Imbolc brings us the first glimmer of spring, the Earth is beginning to stir from Her long winter's sleep. It is a time for new beginnings, and many of us cleanse and purify our homes and sacred spaces in preparation for Spring.

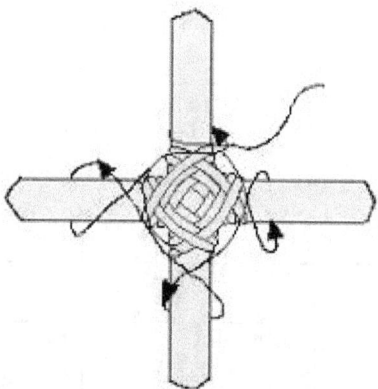

**For practitioners of sacred healing, it is considered prudential to keep the Imbolc Rowan Cross Protection Charm in their vicinity (or at least a picture) to ensure protection from the evil eye.**

The Imbolc Rowan Cross tells us to bring out the sage smudges, floor washes, incense, moon water, brooms, dusters, and mops!  Open the doors, open the windows, out with the old and in with the new!

Once purified you may now create a Rowan twig charm to protect your home or sacred space.

http://sacredwicca.jigsy.com

# **Conclusion**

Most of us would agree that Naturopathy comes to the fore when all else has failed and there seems to be nothing to lose while trying it out. Though miracles do take place, this attitude also leads us to high expectations, unfortunately at an advanced stage of illness.

A backlash of negative feedback is the outcome when Naturopathy is unable to counter the affliction alongwith a feeling of being conned.

With the profusion of unscrupulous charlatans on the web, even Naturopathy is not immune to their skills in promising you the moon and leaving you high and dry after sucking out your life's savings.

The best way to counter this is to exercise due prudence with a discerning eye and take the first step cautiously and determinedly as an experiment. Science and faith will do the rest.

Though mysticism has been kept out of this essay, it may be recalled that Greek temples are replete with tales of vestal virgins assisting in the formal and public religious ceremonies.

There were also many rites which were open to and known only by the initiated who performed them, the most famous example being the Mysteries of Eleusis. In these closed groups, members believed that certain activities healed while also imparting spiritual benefits, amongst them a better after-life.

# References

The Healing Power of the Sacred Woman: Health, Creativity, and Fertility for the Soul by Christine R. Page MD, Bear & Co (November 20, 2012)

The Art of Female Ejaculation – Lisa S. Longhofer, E-BOOK, March 15, 2010

Gray's Anatomy

Wikipedia